Study Guide to accompany

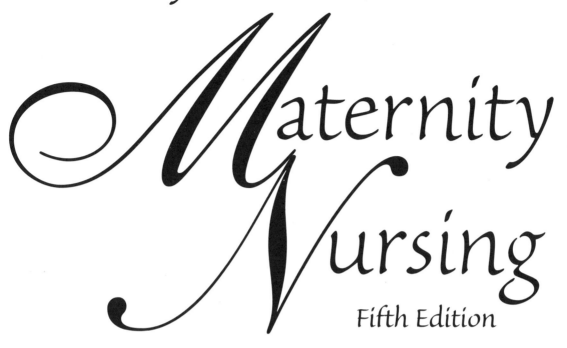

Maternity Nursing

Fifth Edition

Deitra Leonard Lowdermilk, RNC, PhD, FAAN
Shannon E. Perry, RN, PhD, FAAN
Irene M. Bobak, RN, PhD, FAAN

Prepared by
Karen A. Piotrowski, RNC, MSN
Assistant Professor of Nursing
D'Youville College
Buffalo, New York

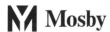 Mosby

A Harcourt Health Sciences Company

St. Louis   London   Philadelphia   Sydney   Toronto

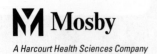

Publisher: **Sally Schrefer**
Editor: **Michael S. Ledbetter**
Developmental Editor: **Laurie K. Muench**
Project Manager: **Gayle May Morris**
Manufacturing Manager: **Donald Carlisle**

FIFTH EDITION

Mosby, Inc.
11830 Westline Industrial Drive
St. Louis, MO 63146

Library of Congress Cataloging-in-Publication Data
Maternity nursing/[edited by] Deitra Leonard Lowdermilk, Shannon E. Perry, Irene M.
  Bobak.—5th ed.
        p.   cm.
Includes bibliographic references and index.
ISBN 0-323-00215-3
1. Maternity nursing.   2. Pediatric nursing.   I. Lowdermilk, Deitra Leonard.
II. Perry, Shannon E.   III. Bobak, Irene M.
[DNLM: 1. Maternal-Child Nursing.   2. Obstetric Nursing.   WY
157.3M4266   1999]
RG951.B66   1999
610.73' 678–dc21
DNLM/DLC
                                                                        98-33732

    00   01   02   03 / 9 8 7 6 5 4 3 2

Contents

INTRODUCTION

This Study Guide is designed to accompany the 5th edition of *Maternity Nursing*. It includes Chapter Review Activities and Critical Thinking Exercises for each chapter in the textbook.

I. *Chapter Review Activities* focus upon **recall** of critical concepts and essential terminology. These activities are designed to help you to identify the important concepts of the chapter and to test your level of knowledge and understanding after reading the chapter. Completion of the activities will provide you an excellent resource for review and will help you to develop the theoretical foundation necessary to answer the critical thinking exercises which follow, enabling you to pass both course and the NCLEX-RN examinations and to manage the care of your patients in the clinical setting. Answers to the activities or answer guidelines are provided in the **Answer Key** located at the end of this guide.

II. *Critical Thinking Exercises* focus upon **application** of critical chapter concepts. These exercises present typical patient care situations, requiring you to apply concepts found in the chapter to solve problems, make decisions concerning care management, and provide responses to a patient's questions and concerns. The exercises may be completed on your own or with members of your study group. Completing the critical thinking exercises will help you prepare for clinical experiences, course examinations, and the NCLEX-RN examination, all of which focus on problem-solving and application of nursing knowledge. Guidelines for completing the exercises and the specific section, subsection, table, and/or box where content can be found are provided in the **Answer Key** located at the end of this guide.

MERLIN: *MATERNITY NURSING,* *5TH EDITION* WEB SITE

Throughout the textbook are references to the Web address for the Lowdermilk: *Maternity Nursing, 5th Edition* home page. This site provides information about the text, biosketches about the authors, links to related Mosby titles and WebLinks, and special related sections for students, clinicians, and faculty.

Specially designed to accompany the textbook are the Student Station, the Faculty Forum, and the Clinician's Corner. These are locations where special information is posted and where users of the text may communicate with Mosby and the authors. The Student Station and the Faculty Forum contain sections on "Teaching Tips", "Content Updates", and "New WebLinks" that have been located and posted. Additionally, faculty using the text have the opportunity at these sites to ask questions and post teaching tips they have found useful. These tips are then reviewed by the authors and posted for all users to access. Finally, the Faculty Forum contains links to Mosby author guidelines, reviewer and contributor inquiry forums, and a location where faculty may bring their ideas for publication.

WEBLINKS

A new feature to accompany *Maternity Nursing, 5th Edition* is WebLinks, which brings the textbook alive by permitting students to access new information located on the Internet as well as to participate in multi-media learning. Each identified Web site has been selected to reinforce and/or supplement materials in the text. An off-site developer has created and posted each site. Although each site has been screened for appropriateness to the content of the textbook, Mosby is not responsible for the content of the Web sites. The sites are continuously scanned for updates and changes in url addresses.

GETTING TO THE WEBLINKS

WebLinks are mentioned throughout the textbook. Also, inside the front cover of the textbook, opposite the title page, is a pull-off tab with a passcode number. Instructors and students will need to register at the designated Web site before accessing WebLinks pages.

To directly access WebLinks, the user must have an Internet account. For convenience, Mosby has included AT&T Internet software on the free CD-ROM that accompanies the textbook. Persons without Internet access may choose to subscribe for service using AT&T software or another Internet provider of their choice.

WHAT IS AVAILABLE AT THE WEBLINKS SITE?

Once registered at the textbook home page, the use is able to access WebLinks. The links have been organized to parallel the table of contents of the textbook. When the user double-clicks on the table-of-content headings (chapter titles), a second screen appears with the WebLinks addresses. Double-clicking on any of the annotated WebLinks addresses will take the use directly to the Web site. The contents of the WebLinks sites are the property of the individual developers or organizations. Mosby has made no attempt to modify or screen the materials except for their relevance to the subject matter in the textbook.

We hope that users will share addresses of additional appropriate sites located while "cruising" the Internet so that we can post them for other users. These can be e-mailed to Mosby at the designated area on the textbook home page.

MOSBY'S ELECTRONIC IMAGE COLLECTION
TO ACCOMPANY *MATERNITY NURSING, 5TH EDITION*

Now available to accompany the textbook is Mosby's Electronic Image Collection, containing electronic versions of over 100 photographs and illustrations from the text to assist in lecture and classroom presentations. Each image may be selected from the CD-ROM and imported into a Power Point presentation or printed to a paper hard copy or transparency acetate. Complete instructions for use of the electronic image collection and a list of the figure numbers and legends are provided in the pamphlet packaged with the CD-ROM.

CHAPTER 1

Contemporary Maternity Nursing

Chapter Review Activities

Matching

Match the definition in Column I with the appropriate descriptive term in Column II.

COLUMN I

- _C_ 1. Number of live births in one year per 1,000 population
- _H_ 2. Infant whose age at birth is less than 38 weeks gestation
- _D_ 3. Number of women who die as a result of births and complications of pregnancy, childbirth, and the puerperium (the first 42 days after termination of the pregnancy) per 100,000 live births
- _E_ 4. Number of stillbirths and the number of neonatal deaths per 1,000 live births
- _A_ 5. Number of births per 1,000 women between the ages of 15 and 44 (inclusive), calculated on a yearly basis
- _G_ 6. Infant whose weight at birth is less than 2,500 g (5 pounds, 8 ounces)
- _B_ 7. Number of deaths during the first year of life per 1,000 live births
- _F_ 8. Number of deaths during the first 28 days of life per 1,000 live births

COLUMN II

- A. Fertility rate
- B. Infant mortality rate
- C. Birth rate
- D. Maternal mortality rate
- E. Neonatal mortality rate
- F. Perinatal mortality rate
- G. Low-birth-weight infant
- H. Preterm infant

Fill in the Blanks

Insert the term that corresponds to each of the following definitions.

9. _Maternitng_ Specialty area of nursing practice that focuses on the care of childbearing women and their families through all stages of pregnancy and childbirth, as well as the first four weeks after birth.

10. _____ Practice that is based on findings obtained through research and clinical trials.

11. _____ Method of care that measures effectiveness of care against benchmarks or standards based on results achieved by others. Quality indicators include _____, _____, and _____.

12. _____ A method of guiding care for a patient that focuses on meeting the patient's needs while promoting efficiency and cost-effectiveness.

13. _____ An approach to health care that emphasizes self-help and assuming responsibility for wellness. The patient is expected to seek information and to take an active role in his/her health care.

14. _____Guidelines for nursing practice based on current knowledge and representative of levels of practice agreed on by leaders in the specialty area of nursing. These guidelines are dynamic and change overtime to reflect changes in nursing practice, society, and the health-care system.

15. _____Umbrella term for the use of communication technologies and electronic information to provide or support health care when the participants are separated by distance.

16. Identify the factors that contribute to infant mortality in the United States.

17. State three major changes that have occurred in childbirth practices and describe how each change has affected the quality of health care.

18. List the most common barriers to early and ongoing prenatal care in the United States.

True or False

Circle "T" if true or "F" if false for each of the following statements. Correct the false statements.

T **F** 19. The neonatal period refers to the first month of an infant's life.

T **F** 20. Currently the highest birth rates are for women between 20 and 29 years of age.

T **F** 21. An abortion refers to the expulsion or removal of an embryo or fetus from the uterus at 15 weeks gestation or less, weighing 750 gm or less, or measuring 20 cm or less.

T **F** 22. Births to unmarried women are frequently related to less favorable outcomes because there are typically a large number of adolescents in this group.

T F 23. One fourth of all births in the United States are to unmarried women, with the highest rate among African-American women.

T F 24. Infant mortality can be reduced by shifting the emphasis from high technology to improving access to preventive health-care services, especially for low-income families.

T F 25. The greatest risk for giving birth to a low birth-weight infant occurs among Hispanic women.

T F 26. The United States ranks 20th for infant mortality among industrialized nations and relates to inadequate access to prenatal care and socioeconomic barriers for child-bearing women.

T F 27. Maternal mortality is a common indicator of the adequacy of prenatal care and the health of the nation as a whole.

T F 28. Maternal mortality for African-American women is four times higher than Caucasian women.

T F 29. Younger women (under 20 years of age), especially those belonging to a minority group, are less likely to seek and receive early, ongoing prenatal care when they are pregnant.

T   F   30. The most significant barrier to accessible prenatal care is the inability to pay.

T   F   31. The number of pregnant women beginning prenatal care during their first trimester has increased.

T   F   32. The number of multiple births has increased, most likely related to childbearing at an early age and the use of fertility drugs.

T   F   33. The incidence of high-risk pregnancies has steadily decreased since 1990.

Critical Thinking Exercises

1. Imagine that you are the nursing director of an inner city prenatal clinic that serves a large number of minority women, many of whom are younger than 20 years. Describe five nursing services you would provide for these women that would help to reduce the potential for infant and maternal morbidity and mortality, and low birth weight. Utilize the biostatistical data and risk behaviors presented in this chapter to support the types of services you propose.

2. Support the accuracy of the following statement: An emphasis on high-technology medical care and life-saving techniques will not reduce the rate of preterm and low birth-weight infants in the United States.

3. Propose three changes in health care and its delivery that you believe will improve the health status and well being of mothers and their infants and reduce the rate of infant and maternal mortality. Support your answer by using the content presented in Chapter 1 and your own experiences with the health-care system.

4. Self-care approaches in health-care management are appealing to women who want to assume responsibility for their own level of wellness and to become active partners with their health-care providers. Discuss the care measures that you, as a nurse, would implement when providing maternal health care to enhance a pregnant woman's responsibility for herself and partnership with you.

CHAPTER 2

The Family and Culture

Chapter Review Activities

Matching

Match the family described in Column I with the appropriate family form from Column II.

COLUMN I

_B_ 1. Miss Manning lives with her 4-year-old adopted Korean daughter, Kim.

_B_ 2. Anne and Duane are married and live with their daughter, Susan, and Duane's mother, Ruth.

_D_ 3. Gloria and Andy are a married couple living with their new baby girl, Annie.

_C_ 4. Carl and Allan are a gay couple living with Carl's daughter, Sally, whom they are raising together.

___ 5. The Smith family consists of Jim, his second wife, Jane, and Jim's two daughters by a previous mariage.

___ 6. Laurie and John have been divorced for three years. They share custody of their four children.

COLUMN II

A. Binuclear family

B. Single parent family

C. Homosexual family

D. Nuclear family

E. Extended family

F. Reconstituted (blended) family

Fill in the Blanks

Insert the cultural concept that most accurately reflects each of the following descriptions.

7. Mrs. Mendez, a Mexican-American woman with a newborn, tells the nurse not to include certain foods on her meal tray since her mother told her to avoid those foods while breast-feeding. The nurse tells her that she doesn't have to avoid any foods and should eat whatever she desires. _____.

8. Ms. Pham, an immigrant from Vietnam, has lived in the United States for one year. She tells you that she enjoys wearing blue jeans and sneakers on casual occasions like shopping, even though she never would have done so in Vietnam. _____.

9. A Cambodian family immigrated to the United States and have been living in Denver for more than 5 years. The parents express concern about their children aged 10, 13, and 16, stating, "The children act so differently now. They are less respectful to us, want to eat only American food, and go to rock concerts. It's hard to believe they are our children." _____.

10. The Amish represent an important ethnic community located in Lancaster, Pennsylvania. _____.

11. The nurse is preparing a healthy diet plan for Mrs. Ostrowski. In doing so, she takes the time to include the Polish foods that are familiar to Mrs. Ostrowski. _____.

12. A set of guidelines an individual follows as a member of a particular social group that tells the person how to view the world and how to relate to other people, supernatural forces, and the natural environment. _____.

13. A central concern of nurses is to plan and provide care that reflects and respects the values and guidelines a patient adheres to as a member of a particular social group. _____.

14. A nursing practice approach that focuses on the way people of different cultures perceive life events and the health-care system. _____.

Insert the term that corresponds to each of the following definitions related to family theory.

15. _____ Essential family activities related to _____, _____, _____, _____, and _____. These interdependent activities depend on the physical and mental health of family members and are influenced by cultural beliefs, values, and sentiments.

16. _____ Interactive processes that allow family members to perform essential activities by working cooperatively with each other and assuming appropriate social roles. Family members use _____ to determine roles and role responsibilities. _____ are set up by a family between itself and society. A family sets up _____ through which it interacts with society and ensures that its members receive their share of resources.

17. _____ A family theory based on a science of wholeness that is characterized by interaction among the components of the family and between the family and the environment. The family is viewed as a whole that is different from the sum of the individual members.

18. _____ A family theory that focuses on the family as it moves in time. Each family member progresses along phases of growth, from dependence through active independence, and to interdependence. The family structure and function also vary over time.

19. _____ A family theory that is concerned with the ways families react to stressful events and suggests factors that promote adaptation to these events. The way a family responds and adapts is influenced by the stressor itself, the family's existing resources, and the family's perception of the stressor. Stress must be studied within the _____ and _____ contexts in which the family is living.

True or False

Circle "T" if true or "F" if false for each of the following statements. Correct the false statements.

T F 20. Cultural beliefs and practices related to childbearing and parenting for a subculture must be assessed for each woman and family representing that subculture because variations in beliefs and practices are possible.

T F 21. Women from Southeast Asia often vocalize while experiencing the pain and discomfort associated with the childbirth process.

T F 22. African-American women seek prenatal care early since they view pregnancy as a time when women require medical care and supervision.

T F 23 Hispanic women appreciate the opportunity to shower or bathe as soon as possible after birth.

T F 24. The nurse should recognize that a Vietnamese woman may not wish to breastfeed until her milk comes in because she believes that newborns should not be fed colostrum since it is dirty.

T F 25. European and American women typically prefer a technology-dominated childbirth approach rather than a natural approach.

T F 26. Native-American women often use herbal concoctions to promote uterine contractions during labor and to stop bleeding in the postpartum period.

T F 27. Hispanic-American women often desire and expect reduced activity or even bed rest for as long as three days after birth.

28. List the five categories of family functions and identify specfic family activities representative of each category.

29. Discuss the maternity nursing implications for each of the following family theories:
    A. Family systems theory

    B. Family developmental theory

30. Discuss why the nurse should take each of the following "products of culture" into consideration when providing care within a cultural context.
    A. Communication

    B. Space

    C. Time

    D. Family roles

31. Nurses must avoid making stereotypical assumptions when caring for patients from specific sociocultural or religious groups. Identify the factors that influence the degree to which a woman and her family adhere to their subculture's traditional beliefs and practices related to childbearing and parenting.

Multiple Choice Questions

Circle the one correct option and state the rationale for the option chosen.

32. A gay couple is raising the son of one of the men. The nurse caring for this family should recognize that
    A. The son has an increased likelihood of being gay himself
    B. Research indicates that children of homosexual parents appear to grow and thrive as well as children in heterosexual families
    C. The son will have difficulty developing a sexual relationship with a female partner
    D. The gay and lesbian family form is rare in the United States

33. A family with open boundaries
    A. Uses available support systems to meet its needs
    B. Is more prone to crisis related to increased exposure to stressors
    C. Discourages family members from setting up channels
    D. Strives to maintain family stability by avoiding outside influences

34. Families in the launching stage of the family life cycle are involved in accomplishing which of the following developmental tasks?
    A. Establishing financial independence
    B. Negotiating tasks related to childrearing and household maintenance
    C. Renegotiating the marital relationship as a dyad
    D. Maintaining own and/or couple functioning and interests in face of physiologic decline

35. Which one of the following nursing actions is most likely to reduce a client's anxiety and enhance the patient's personal security as it relates to the concept of personal space needs?
    A. Touching the patient before and during procedures
    B. Providing explanations when performing tasks
    C. Making eye contact as much as possible
    D. Reducing the need for the patient to make decisions

36. A Native-American woman gave birth to a baby girl 12 hours ago. The nurse notes that the woman keeps her baby in the bassinet except for feeding and states that she will wait until she gets home to begin breastfeeding. The nurse recognizes this behavior as a reflection of
   A. Embarrassment
   B. Delayed attachment
   C. Disappointment that the baby is a girl
   D. Her belief that babies should not be fed colostrum

Crossword Puzzle

The Family and Culture

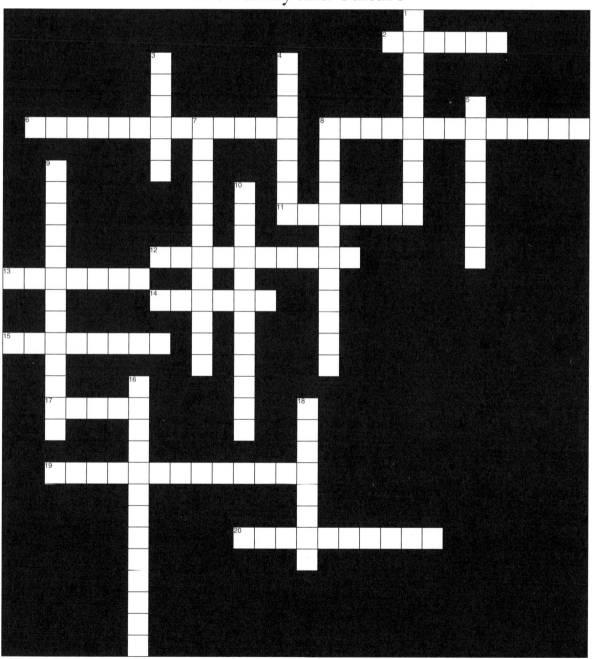

Across

2. Practices and behaviors that are characteristic of a culture and provide a sense of constancy with the culture's heritage.

6. Process in which a family integrates children into society and transfers values relating to behavior, tradition, language, religion, and prevailing or previous social moral attitudes.

8. _____ theory views the family as a complex of elements in mutual interaction. (2 words)

11. A set of guidelines that tells members of a particular social group how to view the world and how to relate to other people, supernatural forces, and the natural environment.

12. Recognizing that people from different cultural backgrounds actually see the same situation differently reflects the concept of cultural _____.

13. Family group, consisting of parents and their dependent children, that lives apart from the parents', family of origin, and is usually economically independent.

14. Families with a _____-oriented sense of time are more likely to return for follow-up visits related to health care.

15. A family form that includes the nuclear family and other blood-related people (kin) such as grandparents, aunts, uncles, and cousins.

17. Dimensions of personal _____ comfort zones and feelings of territoriality are developed within a cultural setting. Actions such as touching the patient, placing the patient in proximity to others, taking away personal possessions, and making decisions for the patient affect the need for distance and can thereby decrease personal security and heighten anxiety.

19. Changes that take place in one or both groups when people from different cultures come in contact with one another and exchange and adopt each other's mannerisms, styles, and practices.

20. The function of a family that is met by the provision of physical necessities such as food, clothing, and shelter.

Down

1. A group existing within a larger cultural system that retains its own characteristics.

3. Composed of two or more people who are joined together by bonds of sharing and emotional closeness.

4. Determining the allocation of resources with a budget and ensuring financial security of family members reflects this family function.

5. Through family _____, family members assume appropriate social roles to accomplish the required family functions.

7. Process in which one cultural group loses its identity and becomes a part of the dominant culture.

8. _____ theory is also know as the ABCX theory. It describes how families experiencing the same stressor may adapt differently to that event based upon the stressor itself, the family's existing resources, and the family's perception of the stressor. (2 words)

9. Being centered in one's own cultural system, judging the world in general by the standards established in that particular system. It is the view that one's cultural way of doing things is the right and natural way—my group is the best.

10. Families that have a _____-_____ sense of time strive to maintain tradition and have little motivation for formulating future goals. (2 words)

16. Family _____ theory views the family as it moves through time. The family demonstrates variations in structure and function, passes through a variety of stages, and accomplishes specific tasks as it progresses through the family life cycle.

18. While families establish boundaries between themselves and society, they also set up _____ through which they interact with society and ensure that they receive their share of social resources.

Critical Thinking Exercises

1. Imagine that you are a nurse working in a clinic that provides prenatal services to a multicultural community predominated by Hispanic, African-American, and Asian families. Describe how you would adapt care measures to reflect the cultural beliefs and practices of pregnant women and their families from each of the following cultural groups.
   Hispanic

   African-American

   Asian

2. Pamela is a 20-year-old Native-American woman. She is 3 months pregnant and has come to the prenatal clinic on the reservation where she lives for her first visit to obtain some prenatal vitamins that her friends at work told her are important.

   A. State the questions the nurse should ask to determine Pamela's cultural explanations about childbearing.

   B. Describe the communication approach the nurse would consider when interviewing Pamela.

   C. Identify the Native-American beliefs and practices regarding childbearing that may influence Pamela's approach to her pregnancy and birth.

3. A nurse has been providing care to the Martinez family. This family recently experienced the birth of twin girls at 38 weeks gestation. It is the first birth experience for both parents and the first grandchildren for the extended family. Both newborns are healthy and living at home.

   A. Identify the family life stage being experienced by this family.

   B. State the developmental tasks that this family needs to accomplish.

   C. Describe the Hispanic cultural beliefs and practices that the Martinez family might use as guidelines to provide care to their twin girls.

4. The nurse-midwife at a prenatal clinic has been assigned to care for a refugee couple from Bosnia who have recently immigrated to the United States. The woman has just been diagnosed as 2 months pregnant. Neither she nor her husband speaks English. Outline the process that this nurse should use when working with a translator to facilitate communication with this couple, thereby enhancing care management.

CHAPTER 3

Community and Home Care

Chapter Review Activities

True or False

Circle "T" if true or "F" if false for each of the following statements. Correct the false statements.

T F 1. It is anticipated that by the year 2000 the hospital will assume a greater role in the care of pregnant women, their newborns, and families.

T F 2. Infant mortality is a statistic widely used to compare the health status of different populations.

T F 3. The rate of reported child abuse and neglect has begun a slow but steady decline.

T F 4. Mortality or death rates are calculated on the number of deaths attributed to a particular health problem such as lung cancer per 100,000 population.

T F 5. Breast self-examination is an example of secondary prevention.

T F 6. Immunization programs are an example of tertiary prevention.

T F 7. The majority of homeless families (53%) are headed by young, single women.

T F 8. Pregnant women who are homeless may have more difficulty with the normal discomforts of pregnancy, resulting in an increased dependence on drugs if they are addicted.

T F 9. Migrant laborers are considered to be episodically homeless since their shelter often depends on seasonal employment.

T F 10. Most migrant laborers value their health and readily seek health-promotion and disease-prevention services.

T F 11. Refugees typically come to the United States for economic reasons.

T F 12. The perinatal continuum of care starts with family planning and preconception care and ends when the infant is 1 year of age.

T F 13. Home health care became a viable health-care alternative when third-party payers pushed for cost containment in maternity services.

T F 14. A proprietary home-care perinatal service is considered to be a nonprofit agency.

T F 15. Women who require bed rest or intravenous fluids during their pregnancies must be hospitalized and therefore are not candidates for home care.

T F 16. Infection control measures are less important when care is given in the patient's home.

T F 17. When documenting a home visit, the nurse should avoid statements such as "no change" or "same as last visit."

Fill in the Blanks

Insert the term that corresponds to each of the following descriptions.

18. Most definitions of community share three characteristics, namely _____, _____, and _____.

19. _____ who reside in a community make up its core. They are influenced by the subsystems of the community, namely _____, _____, _____, _____, _____, _____, and _____.

20. _____ is collected every 10 years. Information is gathered regarding _____, _____, _____ and _____ distribution, _____ status, _____ level, _____, and _____ characteristics.

21. Analyzing individual census tracts helps to identify subpopulations or _____, with differing needs.

22. _____ includes efforts made before the development of illness to promote general health and well-being. It also includes specific protection, such as _____ or _____.

23. _____ involves early detection of health problems so that treatment can begin before significant disability occurs. This includes various methods of _____.

24. _____ is the treatment and rehabilitation of persons who have developed diseases.

25. _____ are groups of people who are at higher risk of developing physical, mental, or social health problems or who are more likely to have worse outcomes from these health problems than the population as a whole. These groups often include the _____, _____, _____, and _____.

26. A committee of experts from many community health-related organizations has identified a set of indicators that can be used to assess the health and well-being of a community.
    A. List the indicators of health status outcome.

    B. List the indicators of risk factors.

27. Identify five special population groups that are more vulnerable than the general population to reproductive health risks.

28. Cite the social and health problems faced by migrant laborers and their families.

29. State three characteristics of refugees that can significantly increase the difficulties they experience.

30. Identify the factors that make home care a growth area for perinatal services.

31. Describe the ways that nurses can provide care to perinatal patients using the telephone.

32. State the advantages and disadvantages of perinatal home visits.

33. Identify the safety and infection control issues home-care nurses must consider when preparing for and conducting a home visit.

Critical Thinking Exercises

1. For a nurse working in home care, it would be helpful to become familiar with the neighborhood and resources in which her or his patients interact.
   A. Describe the Windshield Survey.

B. Discuss how the nurse could use the findings from this survey to provide health care to patients who reside in the assessed community.

2. Marie is a single parent of two young children aged 4 and 1 year. She and her children have been homeless for 3 months since her husband abandoned her and she lost her job because she had no one to help her care for her children.

A. Discuss the types of health problems to which Marie and her children are most vulnerable.

B. Research indicates that Marie is at increased risk for becoming pregnant again. State the factors that make Marie more vulnerable.

C. Outline the principles that should guide a nurse in providing care to Marie and her children if they seek health care at the homeless shelter's clinic.

3. Consuelo is the wife of a migrant laborer. She and her husband, along with their two children, have been working on a California farm for two weeks. She has arrived at a health center established for migrant laborers and has stated that she is four months pregnant. As the woman's health nurse practitioner assigned to care for Consuelo, what approaches would you use to ensure that Consuelo obtains quality health care that addresses her unique health risks as a migrant worker?

4. Write a series of questions that you would ask when making a postpartum follow-up call to a woman who gave birth three days ago.

5. You have been assigned to make a home visit to a postpartum woman who gave birth 36 hours ago.

   A. Outline the approach you would take in preparing for this visit.

   B. Describe your actions during the visit using the care management process as a format.

   C. Discuss how you would end the visit.

   D. Identify important postpartum visit interventions.

6. Angela has been diagnosed recently with hyperemesis gravidarum and has been hospitalized to stabilize her fluid and electrolyte balance. The hospital-based nurse must evaluate Angela for referral to home care.

   A. State the criteria that this nurse should follow to determine Angela's readiness for discharge from hospital to home care.

   B. Angela has been discharged and will be receiving parenteral nutrition in her home. Discuss the additional information required related to high-technology home care.

   C. Identify specific home environment criteria that must be met to ensure the safety and effectiveness of Angela's treatment.

CHAPTER 4

Health Promotion and Prevention

Chapter Review Activities

1. Preconception care has become an integral component of perinatal health care.
   A. Describe the concept of preconception care, including its importance in achieving the goal of a healthy and positive pregnancy outcome for the parents, newborn, and family.

   B. List the purposes of preconception care and counseling.

   C. State the components of preconception care.

   D. Identify the individuals who should participate in this type of health-care service.

2. Identify the most common reasons why women seek health care.

True or False

Circle "T" for true or "F" for false for each of the following statements. Correct each of the false statements.

T F 3. Preconception care and counseling is a health-care service designed primarily for women of childbearing age who have chronic health problems.

T F 4. More than 50% of pregnancies in the United States each year are unintended.

T F 5. Approximately 30% of couples in the United States experience some degree of infertility.

T F 6. The mean age for menopause is 60 years.

T F 7. During the climacteric, women should continue to use birth control since pregnancy can still occur.

T F 8. Women tend to use primary care services more often than men and do so more effectively.

T F 9. Women older than 35 years of age experience a different physical response to pregnancy than women who are younger.

T F 10. Smoking increases the risk for osteoporosis after menopause.

T F 11. Women are more likely than men to abuse drugs.

T F 12. Maternal cocaine use is the leading cause of fetal mental retardation in the United States.

T F 13. Birth defects have been related to moderate to high caffeine consumption.

T F 14. The choice of contraception has no impact on the risk for contracting a sexually transmitted disease.

T F 15. In the United States, Caucasian women have the highest rate of cervical cancer.

T F 16. The most common malignancy of the female reproductive system is endometrial cancer.

T F 17. Women are victims of abuse at a rate much greater than men.

T F 18. Race, religion, social background, age, and educational level are significant factors in identifying and differentiating women at risk for abuse.

T F 19. The key feature to establish rape is the absence of consent: threat or coercion implies the lack of consent.

T F 20. It is recommended that a woman's first Pap smear take place at the age of 18 or when she becomes sexually active.

T F 21. Clinical breast examination by a health-care provider is recommended every year for women after the age of 30.

T F 22. The best time to perform breast self-examination (BSE) for women experiencing menstrual periods would be at the end of each period.

T F 23. The American Cancer Society recommends an annual mammogram beginning at age 38.

T F 24. The American Cancer Society recommends yearly Pap smears for all women.

T F 25. It is recommended that dietary fat intake be reduced to an average of 30% or less of the total calorie intake, with saturated fats no more than 10% of calories.

T F 26. Swimming improves cardiovascular fitness and helps to prevent osteoporosis.

T F 27. Kegel exercises help to strengthen abdominal and pelvic muscles.

T F 28. Cigarette smoking among adolescents and young adult women is higher than for men.

29. State the major goals of prenatal care.

30. List the components that should be included in well-women's care.

31. Describe what occurs to a woman's body during the climacteric or the perimenopause period.

32. Discuss three barriers to seeking health care that women encounter. Identify one nursing intervention that can be used to help a woman overcome each barrier.

33. State the impact of using each of the following illicit drugs during a woman's pregnancy.
Cocaine

Heroin

Marijuana

Fill in the Blanks
Insert the term that corresponds to each of the following descriptions.

34. _____ is a nutritional disorder in which women have a distorted view of their bodies and, no matter what their weight, perceive themselves as being fat. They undertake _____ and _____. A coexisting _____ usually accompanies this disorder.

35. _____ is a disorder characterized by secret, uncontrolled binge eating alternating with methods to prevent weight gain, namely _____, _____ or _____, _____, _____, and _____.

36. _____, _____, and _____ or _____ are terms applied to a pattern of assaultive and coercive behaviors that include _____, _____, and _____ attacks as well as _____ coercion afflicted by a male partner in a marriage or other heterosexual, significant, intimate relationship. _____ is often a time when violence begins or escalates.

37. According to the cycle of violence concept, battering occurs in _____ cycles. The pattern that occurs begins with a period of _____ leading to the _____, which is then followed by a period of _____ known as the _____ phase.

38. Childhood sexual abuse is defined as any type of sexual exploitation that involves a child younger than _____ years of age at the time of the first molestation, at least a _____ age difference between victim and perpetrator, and a variety of behaviors between victim and perpetrator, that may include _____, _____, _____, _____, _____, and _____, _____, or _____ penetration.

39. _____ is any type of sexual exploitation between blood relatives or surrogate relatives before the victim reaches the age of _____. If a stranger commits sexual abuse it is considered to be _____.

40. _____ is an act of violence rather than a sexual act and in its strictest sense it is the _____ of the female _____ or _____ without the woman's consent. Forms or types of this act of violence include _____, _____, _____, _____, and _____. _____ is a term used to describe an act of force with a much broader definition that includes unwanted or uncomfortable _____, _____, _____, _____, _____ or other _____ acts.

41. List the possible consequences of sexually transmitted infections.

42. Identify the risks for each of the following gynecologic cancers.
    Cervical

    Endometrial

Ovarian

43. Compare and contrast the characteristics of women in abusive relationships with the characteristics of women in nonviolent relationships:
Abusive relationships

Nonviolent relationships

44. List the long-term symptoms or effects experienced by some incest survivors:
Physical symptoms/effects

Psychosocial symptoms/effects

Crossword Puzzle

Women's Health

Complete this puzzle after reading and studying the content in Chapters 4, 5, 6, and 7.

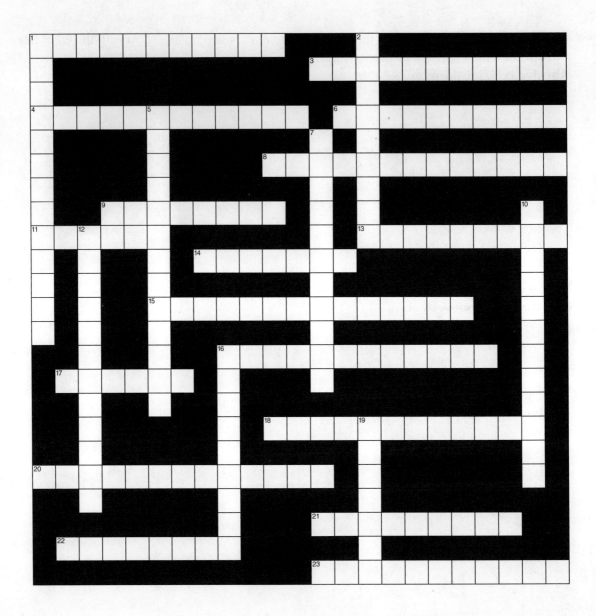

Across

1. Cycle within the menstrual cycle during which the lining of the uterus is shed and then restored.

3. Period in a woman's development during which ovarian function and hormone production declines.

4. Bone loss that occurs during the perimenopausal phase as a result of a decrease in estrogen production.

6. A physical barrier to sperm penetration that also has a chemical action on sperm.

8. Voluntary prevention of pregnancy.

9. Purposeful or spontaneous interruption of pregnancy before 20 weeks gestation.

11. A small T-shaped device that is inserted into the uterine cavity to prevent pregnancy.

13. X-ray of the breast.

14. The entire transitional stage between childhood and sexual maturity.

15. Oxygenated fatty acids classified as hormones that affect smooth muscle contractility and may be involved in dysmenorrhea.

16. Period of uterine bleeding that begins approximately 14 days after ovulation.

17. Thin, stretchable sheath that covers the penis.

18. Intermenstrual bleeding; any episode of bleeding that occurs at a time other than the normal menses.

20. Surgical procedures intended to render the person infertile, most often involving occlusion of the passageways for the ova and sperm.

21. Benign tumors of the smooth muscle of the uterus, also known as fibroids or myomas; they are a common cause of menorrhagia.

22. First menstruation.

23. Excessive menstrual bleeding either in duration or amount.

Down

1. Disorder characterized by the presence and growth of uterine lining tissue outside the uterus.

2. Shallow, dome-shaped rubber device with a flexible wire rim that covers the cervix.

5. _____ care and counseling provide women and their partners with information needed to make decisions about their reproductive future and with the care needed to ensure a positive pregnancy outcome.

7. Inability to become pregnant after one year of unprotected intercourse or to carry a pregnancy to viability .

10. _____ smear is a diagnostic test in which cervical cells are collected and examined for abnormal cell growth that is indicative of carcinogenic conditions, potential or actual.

12. Painful menstruation.

16. Occurrence of the last menstrual period; dated with certainty one year after menstruation ceases.

19. Cycle within the menstrual cycle during which the graafian follicle develops, the oocyte matures, ovulation occurs, and the corpus luteum is formed.

Critical Thinking Exercises

1. Alice and her husband George have just been married. At her annual gynecologic check-up, Alice tells the nurse practitioner that she and her husband plan to get pregnant in about one year. Describe the process that the nurse should follow in providing Alice and George with pre-conception care and counseling.

2. Joyce, a 30-year-old woman, arrives at the women's health clinic and is assigned to a nurse practitioner for care. The nurse notes that Joyce is very nervous and seems embarrassed when she tells the nurse that this is the first time she has ever come for "female care." Describe how the nurse should approach Joyce to ensure quality care that meets Joyce's needs and reduces her level of anxiety and embarrassment.

3. Suzanne is a 15-year-old pregnant adolescent. She plans to live with the 17-year-old father of her baby and raise her child with him. Her parents are angry and are refusing to help her since they disapprove of her pregnancy and her determination to live with her boyfriend without being married.
   A. Discuss the risks Suzanne faces as a pregnant adolescent and expectant parent.

   B. Describe how the nurse should address each of these risks when providing Suzanne and her boyfriend with care.

4. Laura is a 28-year-old pregnant woman at 8 weeks gestation. This is her first pregnancy. During the health history interview, she reveals that she smokes at least ½ pack of cigarettes each day. When discussing this practice with the nurse, Laura states, "My friends smoked when they were pregnant and their babies are okay. In fact, two of them had pregnancies that were a little shorter than expected and they had nice small babies." Describe how the nurse should respond to Laura's comments.

5. As a nurse working at a women's health clinic, you have been assigned to design a health promotion and prevention class for a group of young adult women.
   A. Outline the content you would include in the class and the teaching methodologies you would use when discussing each of the following topics:
   Nutrition

   Exercise

   Health Risk Prevention

   B. During the class, one of the women asks what safer sex means and who needs to use it. Describe how you would respond to her question.

   C. Another woman expresses concern about the increase in violence against women. She states, "One of my friends was raped and a colleague at work was beaten by her boyfriend." Discuss how you would respond to this woman's concern and what you would tell the group about measures they could use to protect themselves from violence and injury.

6. Mary comes to the women's health clinic for her yearly gynecologic check-up. During the health history interview, she tells the nurse that she has just about "reached the end of her rope." Mary cites family and work pressures as the cause.
   A. Identify the physical and emotional effects Mary could experience as a result of her high level of stress.

   B. Describe the stress-management techniques the nurse could recommend to Mary to help her reduce her level of stress and cope with it in a healthy manner.

CHAPTER 5

Health Assessment

Chapter Review Activities

Fill in the Blanks

Insert the term that corresponds to each of the following definitions.

1. _____ Fatty pad that lies over the anterior surface of the symphysis pubis.
2. _____ Two rounded folds of fatty tissue covered with skin that extend downward and backward from the mons pubis; their purpose is to protect the inner vulvar structures.
3. _____ Two flat reddish folds composed of connective tissue and smooth muscle, which are supplied with extremely sensitive nerve endings.
4. _____ Hoodlike covering of the clitoris.
5. _____ Fold of tissue under the clitoris.
6. _____ Thin flat tissue formed by the joining of the labia minora; it is underneath the vaginal opening at the midline.
7. _____ Small structure composed of erectile tissue with numerous sensory nerve endings; it increases in size during sexual arousal.
8. _____ Almond-shaped area enclosed by the labia minora that contains openings to the urethra, Skene's glands, vagina, and Bartholin's glands.
9. _____ Skin-covered muscular area between the fourchette and the anus that covers the pelvic structures.
10. _____ Fibromuscular, collapsible tubular structure that extends from the vulva to the uterus and lies between the bladder and rectum. Its mucosal lining is arranged in transverse folds called _____.
11. _____ Anterior, posterior, and lateral pockets that surround the cervix.
12. _____ Location in the cervix where the squamous and columnar epithelia meet; it is the most common site for neoplastic changes; cells from this site are scraped for the Pap smear.
13. _____ Dome-shaped top of the uterus.
14. _____ Highly vascular lining of the uterus.
15. _____ Layer of the uterus composed of smooth muscles that extend in three different directions.
16. _____ Passageways between the ovaries and the uterus; they are attached at each side of the dome-shaped top of the uterus.
17. _____ Almond-shaped organs located on each side of the uterus; their two functions are _____ and the production of the hormones _____, _____, and _____.

18. A nurse working in women's health care must know the female reproductive systems, including the internal and external structures, the interrelationship of these structures, and their normal characteristics. Label each of the following illustrations as indicated. Describe on a separate sheet of paper the normal characteristics and function of each structure. (Use the figures in Chapter 5 and those found in a physical assessment or anatomy textbook to assist you with the labels and descriptions.)

A. External female genitalia

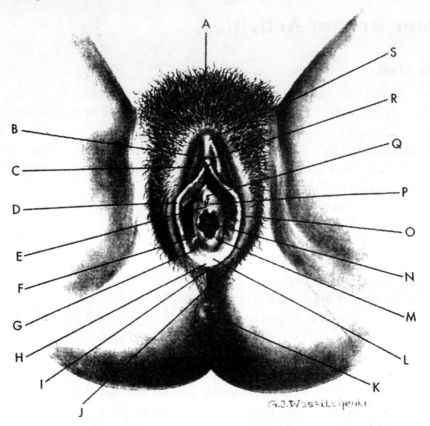

B. Perineal body with surrounding tissues and organs

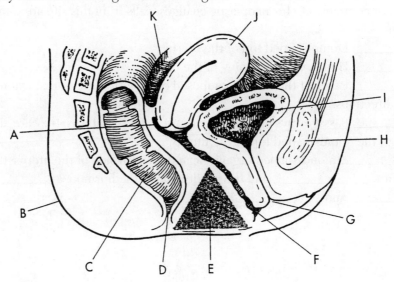

C. Cross section of uterus, adnexa, and upper vagina

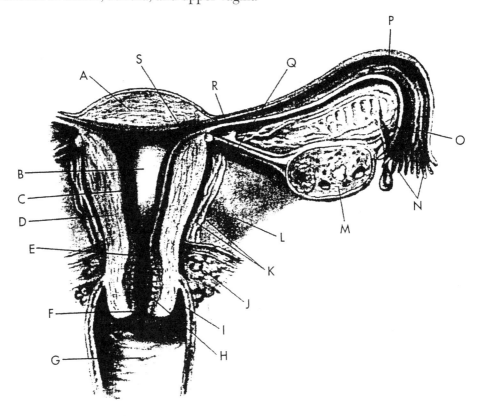

D. Female breast

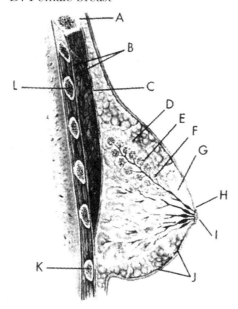

Sagittal section

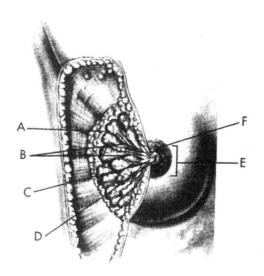

Anterior dissection

E. Female pelvis

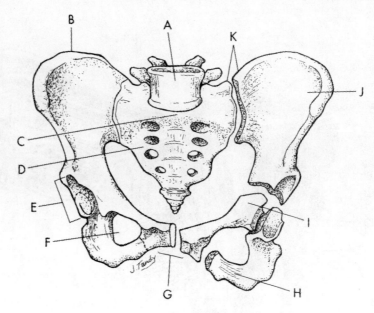

19. The diagram below illustrates the cyclical changes that occur during the menstrual cycle of a woman of childbearing age.

   A. Label the diagram as indicated in terms of hormones, phases and cycles, and specific ovarian structures.

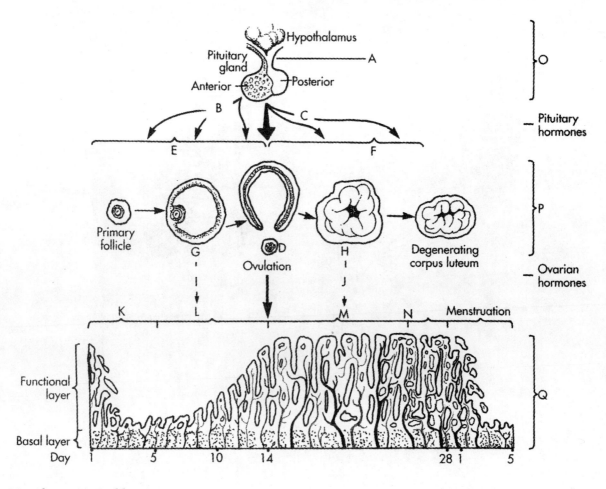

B. Describe the events or changes that occur during each of the following cycles:

Hypothalamic-pituitary cycle

Ovarian cycle

Endometrial cycle

C. Identify cyclical changes that occur in terms of basal body temperature and cervical mucous.

True or False

Circle "T" if true or "F" if false for each of the following statements. Correct the false statements.

T   F   20. Breast swelling, tenderness, and leakage from the nipple are expected assessment findings during the postmenstrual period.

T   F   21. Dysmenorrhea (painful menstruation) is most often associated with the production of estrogen.

T   F   22. Pregnancy is possible at any time after menarche occurs.

T   F   23. Variations in the length of the follicular phase account for almost all variations in the length of menstrual cycles.

T   F   24. Implantation (nidation) of a fertilized ovum usually occurs about 14 days after ovulation.

T   F   25. Mittelschmerz refers to the stretchable quality of cervical mucous that occurs in response to estrogen secretion before ovulation.

T   F   26. Men and women are different in terms of their physiologic response to sexual excitement and orgasm.

T   F   27. The acidity of vaginal secretions is an important body defense against infection.

T   F   28. Vaccination results in passive immunity.

T   F   29. Active immunity is permanent and occurs when colostrum transfers maternal antibodies to the fetus.

T   F   30. For many women, modesty, fear, and anxiety can make the health history interview and the physical examination an ordeal.

T   F   31. Vulvar (genital) self-examination (VSE/GSE) should be performed by all women who are sexually active or 18 years of age or older, at least once a month between menstrual periods.

32. State how each of the following factors can influence the health assessment of women.

Culture

Age

Physical and emotional disorders

Abuse

33. Describe the instructions a woman should be given when she is scheduled for a pelvic examination that will include a Pap smear.

34. Hormones play an important role in the regulation of the menstrual cycle. Describe the function of each of the following hormones:

Gonadotrophin-releasing hormone (Gn-RH)

Follicle-stimulating hormone (FSH)

Luteinizing hormone (LH)

Estrogen

Progesterone

Prostaglandins

35. Complete the following table related to the four phases of the sexual response cycle.

Phase	Reactions common to both sexes	Female reactions	Male reactions
Excitement			
Plateau			
Orgasmic			
Resolution			

Matching

Match the description in Column I with the appropriate term in Column II.

COLUMN I

_____ 36. Study of molecules, cells, organs, and systems responsible for the recognition and disposal of foreign material and how the human body defends itself against this material.

_____ 37. Adaptive form of defensive resistance to infection that occurs if a microorganism overwhelms the body's natural resistance; it allows the body to recognize, remember, and respond to a specific stimulus—an antigen.

_____ 38. Unbroken skin and mucous membranes.

_____ 39. Artificial resistance to infection achieved by infusion of serum or plasma containing high concentration of antibody.

_____ 40. Injection of an antigen that stimulates antibody production and memory without experiencing the disease.

_____ 41. Innate or inborn nonspecific mechanism of the body to resist infection.

_____ 42. Form of resistance to infection that is mediated by the link between T-lymphocytes and phagocytic cells.

_____ 43. Form of resistance that can occur as a result of natural exposure in response to an infection or as a result of injection of an antigen.

_____ 44. Immune system is able to recognize a foreign antigen and build specific antigen-directed antibodies.

COLUMN II

A. First barrier to infection
B. Immunology
C. Natural immunity
D. Acquired immunity
E. Active immunity
F. Vaccination
G. Immunocompetent
H. Passive immunity
I. Cell-mediated immunity

45. Describe each of the following components of the pelvic examination.

External inspection and palpation

Internal examination

Bimanual palpation

Rectovaginal palpation

46. Outline the guidelines that should be followed when performing a Pap smear in terms of each of the following:
Patient preparation

Timing during examination when the specimen is obtained

Sites for specimen collection

Handling of specimens

Frequency of performance

Critical Thinking Exercises

1. Imagine that you are a nurse working at a clinic that provides health care to women. Describe how you would respond to each of the following concerns or questions of women.
   A. Jane, a newly married woman, is concerned that she did not bleed during her first coital experience with her husband. She states, "I was a virgin and always thought you had to bleed when you had sex for the first time. Do you think my husband will still believe I was a virgin on our wedding night?"

B. Andrea is trying to get pregnant. She wonders if there are signs she could observe in her body that would indicate that she is ovulating and therefore able to conceive a baby with her partner.

C. When teaching a group of women, of various ages, about breast self-examination (BSE), they ask you to describe the normal characteristics of the female breast and how these characteristics change as a woman gets older.

D. Anne, a 24-year-old woman asks the nurse about a recommended douche to use a couple of times a week to stay "nice and clean down there."

2. As a nurse working in a women's health clinic, you have been assigned to interview a new female patient to obtain her health history.
   A. Write a series of questions that you would ask to obtain data related to her reproductive and sexual health and practices.

   B. Discuss the therapeutic techniques that you would use to facilitate communication. Give an example of each technique.

3. Self-examinations of the breasts and vulva (genitalia) are important assessment techniques to teach a woman. Outline the procedure that you would use to teach each technique to one of your patients. Include the teaching methodologies that you would use to enhance learning.
   Breast self-examination

Vulvar (genital) self-examination

4. Lu Chen is a 25-year-old exchange student from China who has been living in the United States for 3 months. This is the first time that she is away from home. She comes to the university women's health clinic for a check-up and to obtain birth control. Describe how the nurse assigned to Lu Chen would approach and communicate with her in a culturally sensitive manner.

5. Nurses working in women's health care must be aware of the growing problem of violence against women. All women should be screened when being assessed during health care for the possibility of abuse.
   A. Describe how you, as a nurse, would adjust the environment where the health history interview and physical examination will take place to elicit a woman's confidence and trust.

   B. Identify indicators of possible abuse that you would look for before the appointment and then during the health history interview and physical examination.

   C. State the questions you would ask to screen for abuse.

   D. Discuss the approach you would take if abuse is confirmed during the assessment.

6. As a student you may be assigned to assist a health-care provider during a pelvic examination for one of your patients.
   A. Describe how you would:
   Prepare your patient for the examination

   Support your patient during the examination

   Assist your patient after the examination

   B. Describe how you would assist the health-care provider who is performing the examination.

CHAPTER 6

Common Health Problems

Chapter Review Activities

Fill in the Blanks

Insert the term that corresponds to menstrual disorders for each of the following descriptions.

1. _____ refers to the absence or cessation of menstrual flow. It is a clinical sign of a variety of disorders, but it is most commonly associated with _____. It is also one of the classic signs of _____.

2. _____ or painful menstruation is one of the most common gynecologic problems for women of all ages. Symptoms usually begin with the _____. _____ is a type of painful menstruation that occurs as a result of a physiologic alteration in some women. It usually appears in _____ after menarche once _____ is established since both _____ and _____ are necessary for it to occur. _____ is a type of painful menstruation that is acquired later in life and is associated with pelvic abnormality. Pain often begins _____.

3. _____ is a constellation of physical and psychologic symptoms beginning in the luteal phase of the menstrual cycle. A diagnosis is made only if the following three criteria are met:_____, _____, and _____.

4. _____ is a menstrual disorder that is characterized by the presence and growth of endometrial tissue outside of the uterus. This tissue responds to hormonal stimulation by growing during the _____ and _____ phases of the menstrual cycle and bleeds during or immediately after _____ resulting in an _____ response with subsequent _____ and _____ to adjacent organs. The major symptom of this disorder is _____. Many women also experience bowel symptoms such as _____, _____, and _____. _____ may result from adhesions around the uterus and uterine tubes.

5. _____ is the term used to describe infrequent menstrual periods, whereas _____ refers to scanty bleeding at normal intervals. One of the most common causes of scanty menstrual flow is the use of _____.

6. _____ or _____ refers to any episode of bleeding that occurs other than the normal menses. Causes of this type of bleeding include the use of _____, _____, or _____.

7. _____ or _____ is defined as excessive menstrual bleeding either in duration or amount. The causes may include _____, _____, _____, _____, and _____. _____ are often used to treat this disorder because they increase vasoconstriction and improve platelet aggregation.

8. _____ refers to a wide variety of menstrual irregularities but most often is associated with excessive bleeding of some type. It is most commonly associated with _____ where there is no surge of _____ or if insufficient _____ is produced by the _____ to support the endometrium it will begin to involute and shed. This most often occurs at the _____ when the menstrual cycle is just becoming established at _____ or when it draws to a close at _____. The most common treatment approach is _____ therapy with _____ and _____.

True or False

Circle "T" if true or "F" if false for each of the following statements. Correct the false statements.

T F 9. A pregnancy test is recommended as an initial step when a woman experiences amenorrhea.

T F 10. Premature osteoporosis can occur as a consequence of low levels of progesterone with hypogonadotropic amenorrhea.

T F 11. A woman being treated with hormone replacement therapy for hypogonadotropic amenorrhea is protected from getting pregnant.

T F 12. The exact cause of premenstrual syndrome (PMS) is unknown.

T F 13. When a woman is experiencing primary dysmenorrhea, she should reduce her activity level and avoid exercising for the first 24 hours of this discomfort.

T F 14. Oral contraceptives are the first-line medications for the treatment of primary dysmenorrhea.

T F 15. Endometriosis is a menstrual disorder primarily affecting Caucasian women during their late teens to early twenties.

T F 16. Synarel (nafarelin) is a gonadotrophic-releasing hormone agonist administered at a dose of 200 mg bid by nasal spray to treat endometriosis.

T F 17. The only definitive cure for endometriosis is a total abdominal hysterectomy (TAH) with bilateral salpingooophorectomy (BSO).

T F 18. Aspirin can be used to reduce the size of myomas (fibroids) prior to a myomectomy.

T F 19. Sexually transmitted diseases (STDs) are among the most common health problems in the United States today.

T F 20. The majority of women contracting chlamydia and gonorrhea are 30 years of age or older.

T F 21. Human papillomavirus is the most common and fastest spreading STD in American women today.

T F 22. The VDRL and RPR are used as screening tests for syphilis.

T F 23. Women are the fastest growing population of individuals with human immunodeficiency virus (HIV) infection and acquired immunodeficiency syndrome (AIDS).

T F 24. Once HIV enters the body, seroconversion to HIV positivity usually occurs within 2 to 4 weeks.

T F 25. Presence of HIV antibody in infants younger than 18 months of age is not diagnostic of HIV infection.

T F 26. Standard precautions are to be used once patients have been diagnosed with a bloodborne infection.

T F 27. Fibroadenoma is a rare, benign condition of the breast most commonly seen in middle-aged women.

T F 28. One in ten American women will develop breast cancer in their lifetime.

T F 29. Risk factors help to identity only 25% of women who will eventually develop breast cancer.

T F 30. It is estimated that the majority of breast lumps detected by women are malignant.

T F 31. Lumpectomy and simple, modified, or radical mastectomy have similar 5-year survival and recurrence rates.

32. Hypogonadotropic amenorrhea reflects a problem in the central hypothalamic-pituitary axis.
    A. State the risk factors for this menstrual disorder.

    B. Describe the nurse's role when caring for a woman who has this type of menstrual disorder.

33. List the symptoms that have been associated with PMS.

34. Identify two sexual behaviors that apply to each of the following categories.
    Safest behaviors

    Low-risk behaviors

    Possibly risky (possible exposure) behaviors

High-risk (unsafe) behaviors

35. List the most common sexually transmitted infections in women.

36. Complete the following table related to sexually transmitted infections and vaginal infections.

Infection	Effects	Diagnosis	Management
Chlamydia trachomatis			
Gonorrhea			
Syphilis			
Genital herpes simplex virus			
Human papillomavirus			
Bacterial vaginosis			
Candidiasis			
Trichomoniasis			

Fill in the Blanks

Insert the term that corresponds to pelvic inflammatory disease (PID) for each of the following descriptions.

37. PID is an infectious process that most commonly involves the _____, _____, and more rarely the _____ and _____ surfaces.

38. _____ is estimated to cause _____ of all cases of PID. Most PID results from ascending spread of microorganisms from the _____ and _____ to the _____. This spread most frequently happens at the _____ or following an _____, _____, or _____.

39. Women who have had PID are at increased risk for _____, _____, and _____. Other problems associated with PID include _____, _____, _____, and _____.

40. Signs and symptoms of PID include _____ and one or more of the following: _____, _____, _____, _____, _____, and _____.

41. The most important nursing intervention related to PID is _____ by _____ and _____.

42. Identify factors that place women at risk for contracting a hepatitis B infection.

43. Heterosexual transmission is the most common means of HIV transmission to women.
    A. State the mode of transmission for the HIV.

    B. List the signs and symptoms that may occur during seroconversion to HIV positivity.

    C. Identify the behaviors that place a woman at risk for HIV infection.

D. Outline the care management approach for women who test HIV positive.

44. State two specific precautions for each of the following.
   Standard precautions

   Precautions for invasive procedures

45. List the probable risk factors for breast cancer.

Critical Thinking Exercises

1. Mary, a 17-year-old who experienced menarche at age 16, comes to the women's health clinic for a routine check-up. She complains to the nurse that her last few periods have been very painful. "I have missed a few days of school because of it. What can I do to reduce the pain that I feel during my periods?" Physical examination and testing reveal normal structure and function of Mary's reproductive system. Primary dysmenorrhea is diagnosed.
   A. State one nursing diagnosis that is appropriate for Mary's health problem.

   B. Identify self-care measures the nurse could recommend to address Mary's health problem.

2. Susan has been diagnosed with PMS. Describe the approach the nurse would take in helping Susan deal with this menstrual disorder.

3. Lisa is 26 years old and has been diagnosed recently with endometriosis.
   A. List the signs and symptoms Lisa most likely exhibited to lead to this medical diagnosis.

   B. Lisa asks the nurse, "What is happening to my body as a result of this disease?" Describe the nurse's response.

   C. Lisa asks about her treatment options. "Are there medications I can take to make me feel better?" Describe the action/effect and potential side effects for each of the following pharmacologic approaches to treatment.
   Oral contraceptive pills

   Gonadotrophin-releasing hormone agonists

   Androgenic synthetic steroids

   D. Identify support measures the nurse can suggest to assist Lisa to cope with the effects of endometriosis.

4. Suzanne has just been diagnosed with severe, acute PID as a result of a chlamydia infection. Intravenous antibiotics will be used as the primary medical treatment, followed by oral antibiotics.

   A. Outline a nursing management plan for Suzanne in terms of each of the following.
      Position/activity

      Comfort measures

      Support measures

      Health education

   B. List the recommendations for Suzanne's self-care during the recovery phase.

5. Gloria has tested positive for hepatitis B. Describe the measures the nurse should teach Gloria to implement that decrease the chance of transmission of the virus to other persons in Gloria's life.

6. Sonya is concerned that she has been exposed to HIV and has come to the women's health clinic for testing.

   A. Explain the testing procedure that most likely will be followed to determine Sonya's HIV status.

B. Outline the counseling protocol that should be followed by the nurse caring for Sonya.

7. Molly, a 50-year-old woman, found a lump in her left breast during a breast self-examination. She comes to the women's health clinic for help.
   A. Describe the diagnostic protocol that should be followed to determine the basis for the lump Molly found in her breast.

   B. Molly's lump is diagnosed as cancerous and she elects to have a simple mastectomy based on the information provided by her health-care providers and in consultation with her husband. Describe the nursing care management for each of the following phases of Molly's treatment.
   Preoperative phase

   Immediate postoperative phase

   C. Molly will be discharged within 48 hours after her surgery. Outline the instructions the nurse should give to Molly to prepare her for self-care at home.

   D. Discuss support measures the nurse should use to address the concerns that Molly and her husband will most likely experience and express.

CHAPTER 7

Contraception, Infertility, and Abortion

Chapter Review Activities

True or False: Contraception and Abortion

Circle "T" if true or "F" if false for each of the following statements. Correct the false statements.

T   F   1. Contraception failure rate refers to the percentage of contraceptive users expected to experience an accidental pregnancy during the first year of use, even when they use the method consistently and correctly.

T   F   2. The fertile period extends from 4 days before to 3 to 4 days after ovulation.

T   F   3. When preparing to use the calendar method of periodic abstinence, a woman needs to record accurately the lengths of the previous two menstrual cycles.

T   F   4. Use of nonoxynol 9 with a condom offers some protection against the transmission of sexually transmitted diseases such as gonorrhea, chlamydia, and human immunodeficiency virus.

T   F   5. The female condom may heighten sensation for the man since it is looser than the male condom.

T   F   6. The Norplant system, which consists of six Silastic capsules containing progestin, provides up to 3 years of contraceptive effectiveness.

T   F   7. Norplant thickens cervical mucus and suppresses ovulation completely.

T   F   8. The most common side effect of Norplant is irregular menstrual bleeding.

T   F   9. Use of a diaphragm can increase the risk for urethritis and recurrent cystitis.

T   F   10. The intrauterine device (IUD) is more appropriate than oral contraceptives for women older than 35 years of age and who are heavy smokers.

T   F   11. The copper IUD remains effective for a maximum of 4 years.

T   F   12. Women using combined estrogen and progestin oral contraception should expect heavier menstrual bleeding.

T   F   13. Following a vasectomy, another form of birth control should be used until the sperm count is zero for at least two consecutive semen analyses.

T   F   14. A vasectomy should have no effect on potency, but the volume of ejaculate may be reduced.

T   F   15. No change in hormonal activity or menstrual periods should occur following a tubal ligation.

T   F   16. Phasic oral contraceptive pills provide fixed dosages of both estrogen and progesterone.

T   F   17. Most women having abortions are white, younger than 24 years old, and unmarried.

T   F   18. RU 486 can be taken up to 5 weeks after conception to terminate a pregnancy.

T   F   19. Oxytocin gel or intramuscular injection is the most common medical technique to terminate a pregnancy in the second trimester.

20. State the characteristics of the ideal contraceptive.

21. List the factors that can influence the effectiveness of a contraceptive method.

22. Informed consent is a vital component when helping a woman to choose a contraceptive method that is right for her. The acronym **BRAIDED** is useful in ensuring that all the elements of an informed consent have been met and documented. Indicate the action represented by each letter.

    B

    R

    A

    I

    D

    E

    D

23. June's religious and cultural beliefs prohibit her from using any artificial method of birth control. She is interested in learning about periodic abstinence or natural family planning as a method of contraception. Fill in the blanks in each for the following statements concerning this method.

    A. The two principal problems with periodic abstinence are that the _____ and it is often difficult to _____. Women with _____ have the greatest risk for failure.

    B. Using the calendar method, June and her husband would abstain from day _____ to _____ of her menstrual cycle since her shortest cycle was 23 days and the longest cycle was 33 days.

    C. Basal body temperature (BBT) will _____ about _____ C around the time of ovulation. After ovulation, because of increasing levels of _____, the BBT will _____ about _____ C. This change in BBT will last until _____ before menstruation and is termed the _____. Most counselors recommend abstinence or protected intercourse from the _____ and for _____ of elevated temperature.

    D. The Billings method, also called the _____ method, would require June to recognize and interpret the cyclical changes in the characteristics of her _____ such as _____ and _____.

    E. The Symptothermal method combines _____ and _____ methods with awareness of cycle phase related symptoms such as _____, _____, _____, _____, or _____, and _____.

    F. The Predictor test for ovulation detects the sudden surge of _____ in the urine that occurs approximately _____ hours before ovulation.

24. Alice and Bob use nonprescription chemical and mechanical contraceptive barriers. Label each of the following actions with "C" if correct or "I" if incorrect. Indicate how the action should be changed for those actions labeled "I."

    A. _____ When using a vaginal suppository form of spermicide, Alice waits about 30 minutes after insertion before beginning intercourse.

    B. _____ When using a spermicidal vaginal foam, Alice shakes the container before application.

    C. _____ Alice reapplies the spermicide before each act of intercourse.

    D. _____ Alice douches within 2 hours of intercourse because she finds the spermicidal foam sticky and uncomfortable.

    E. _____ Bob applies a condom over his erect penis leaving an empty space at the tip.

    F. _____ Bob often lubricates the outside of the condom with Vaseline, a petroleum-based lubricant.

    G. _____ Bob uses the same condom if he and Alice repeat intercourse.

25. Joyce has chosen the diaphragm as her method of contraception. Label each of the following actions with "C" if correct or "I" if incorrect. Indicate how the action should be changed for those actions labeled "I."

    A. _____ Joyce came to be refitted after healing was complete following the vaginal birth of her son.

    B. _____ Joyce applies a spermicide only to the rim of the diaphragm just before insertion.

    C. _____ Joyce empties her bladder before inserting the diaphragm.

D. _____ Joyce inserts the diaphragm about 3 to 4 hours before intercourse to increase spontaneity.

E. _____ Joyce applies more spermicide for each act of intercourse.

F. _____ Joyce removes the diaphragm within 1 hour of intercourse.

G. _____ After removal, Joyce washes the diaphragm with warm water and an antiseptic-type soap, dries it, and then applies baby powder.

H. _____ Joyce always uses the diaphragm during her menstrual periods.

26. Cite four factors that can contribute to a woman's decision to seek an induced abortion.

True or False: Infertility

Circle "T" if true or "F" if false for each of the following statements. Correct the false statements.

T   F   27. The traditional definition of infertility is the inability to conceive after at least 1 year of unprotected intercourse.

T   F   28. Infertility that is solely a result of female factors is responsible for approximately 40% to 55% of infertility cases.

T   F   29. Unexplained factors account for 5% to 10% of infertility cases.

T   F   30. Hysterosalpingography, which is scheduled for 2 to 5 days after menstruation, is used to determine tubal patency and to release a blockage if present.

T   F   31. Referred shoulder pain associated with a hysterosalpingogram indicates the presence of an infection in the uterus or the fallopian tubes.

T   F   32. An endometrial biopsy is typically performed late in the menstrual cycle about 2 to 3 days before menstruation is expected to begin.

T   F   33. An increase in scrotal temperature, by using hot tubs and saunas, may adversely affect spermatogenesis.

T   F   34. The use of condoms during genital intercourse for 6 to 12 months will reduce female antibody production in most women who have elevated antisperm antibody titers.

35. Mary and Jim have come for their first visit to the fertility clinic. You must instruct them on the interrelated structures, functions, and processes essential for conception, emphasizing that they are a biologic unit of reproduction.

A. Identify and describe each component required for normal fertility.

B. Support the statement: Assessment of infertility must involve both partners.

36. With some forms of infertility, pharmacologic measures may be effective. Indicate classification, mode of action, contraindications, administration, side effects, and nursing implications including content for health teaching for each of the following medications. Use a drug manual to assist you in gathering this information.

Clomiphene citrate (Clomid, Serophene)

Bromocriptine (Parlodel)

Human menopausal gonadotrophin (Pergonal)

Gonadotrophin-releasing hormone

37. Infertility is considered primary if the woman has _____ or the man has _____. It is considered secondary if the woman has _____. List the probable causes for female and male infertility:

Female infertility   **Male infertility**

Matching

Match the description in Column I with the appropriate test in Column II.

COLUMN I

_____ 38. Immunologic test to determine sperm and cervical mucous interaction.

_____ 39. Examination of the lining of the uterus to detect secretory changes and receptivity to implantation.

_____ 40. Test for adequacy of coital technique, cervical mucus, sperm, and degree of sperm penetration through cervical mucous.

_____ 41. Examination of uterine cavity and tubes using radiopaque contrast material instilled through the cervix.

_____ 42. Examination of pelvic structures by inserting a small endoscope through an incision in the abdominal wall.

_____ 43. Basic test for male infertility

COLUMN II

A. Laparoscopy

B. Postcoital test

C. Endometrial biopsy

D. Hysterosalpingography

E. Sperm immobilization antigen-antibody reaction

F. Semen analysis

44. Alternative birth technologies are being developed and perfected, creating a variety of ethical, legal, financial, and psychosocial concerns.
    A. Define each of the following reproductive alternatives.

    In vitro fertilization (IVF)

    Embryo transfer (ET)

    Gamete intrafallopian transfer (GIFT)

    Zygote intrafallopian transfer (ZIFT)

    Therapeutic intrauterine insemination

    Gestational carrier (embryo host)

    B. Discuss the ethical issues and questions engendered by these alternative technologies.

Critical Thinking Exercises

1. Kathy has come to Planned Parenthood for information on birth control methods and assistance with making her choice. Discuss the approach the nurse should use to help Kathy make an informed decision when choosing contraception that is right for her.

2. June plans to use a combination estrogen-progestin oral contraceptive.
    A. Describe the mode of action for this type of contraception.

    B. List the advantages of using oral contraception.

C. Identify the factors, that if present in June's health history, would constitute absolute or relative contraindications to the use of oral contraception with estrogen and progesterone.

D. Cite the side effects that can occur in terms of the following:
Estrogen excess

Estrogen deficiency

Progestin excess

Progestin deficiency

E. Using the acronym ACHES, identify the signs and symptoms that would require June to stop taking the pill and notify her health-care provider.
A

C

H

E

S

F. Specify the instructions you would give June about taking the pill to ensure maximum effectiveness.

3. Beth has decided to try the cervical cap. Describe the principles that should guide Beth's use of this method to maximize effectiveness and to minimize or prevent complications.

4. Anita has just had a Copper-T 380 A IUD inserted. Specify the instructions you would give to Anita before she leaves the women's health clinic after the insertion.

5. Judy (6 - 4 - 1 - 1 - 3) and Allen, both aged 36, are contemplating sterilization now that their family is complete. They are seeking counseling regarding this decision.
   A. Describe the approach a nurse should use in helping Judy and Allen make the right decision for them.

   B. They decide that Allen will have a vasectomy. Discuss the preoperative and postoperative care and instructions required by Allen.

6. Anne and her husband, Ian, will be using the symptothermal method of natural family planning (NFP).
   A. List the assessment components of this method.

   B. Outline the teaching plan you would use to ensure that Anne and Ian will do the following accurately:
   Measure basal body temperature (BBT)

Evaluate cervical mucus characteristics

C. State the effectiveness of this method of contraception.

7. Mark and his wife, Mary, are undergoing testing for impaired fertility.
   A. List the components of the assessment for both Mary and Mark.
   Assessment for the woman

   Assessment for the man

   B. Mark must provide a specimen of semen for analysis. Describe the procedure he should follow to ensure accuracy of the test.

   C. State the semen characteristics that will be assessed and the values expected for each.

   D. A postcoital test will be part of the diagnostic process for Mary and Mark. Describe the instructions you would give them to maximize the effectiveness and accuracy of the test.

E. Describe nursing support measures that should be used when working with Mark and Mary.

8. Suzanne has been scheduled for a diagnostic laparoscopy to determine the basis of her infertility.
   A. Indicate when this test should be done during the menstrual cycle.

   B. Specify the preoperative measures required to prepare Suzanne for this procedure.

   C. Suzanne asks you why the test is needed and what will be done during the test. Describe your response.

   D. Specify the postoperative care measures required, including the discharge instructions that Suzanne should receive.

9. Edna is a 20-year-old unmarried woman. She is 9 weeks pregnant and is unsure about what to do. She comes to the women's health clinic and asks for the nurse's help in making her decision, stating, "I just cannot support a baby right now. I am alone and trying to finish my education. What can I do?"
   A. Describe the approach the nurse should take in helping Edna to make a decision that is right for her.

   B. Edna elects to have an abortion. A vacuum aspiration will be performed in the morning. Laminaria will be used in preparation for the procedure. Edna asks what will happen to her as part of the abortion procedure. Describe how the nurse should respond to Edna's question.

C. Identify three nursing diagnoses related to Edna's situation and the procedure she is facing.

D. Describe the nursing measures related to the physical care and emotional support that Edna will require as part of this procedure.

E. Outline the discharge instructions that Edna should receive.

CHAPTER 8

Conception and Fetal Development

Chapter Review Activities

Fill in the Blanks

Insert the term that corresponds to the process of conception and implantation for each of the following descriptions.

1. At the time of ovulation, the _____ is released from the ruptured _____. _____ of the uterine tube capture the ovum and propel it through the uterine _____ toward the uterus. Ova are fertile for about _____ hours after ovulation.

2. Following ejaculation, _____ reach the site of fertilization in an average of _____ hours and remain viable in a woman's reproductive system for _____ days. With the process of _____, the protective coating from the sperm heads is removed, allowing _____ to escape. Fertilization occurs in the _____ of the uterine tube. Once penetrated by a sperm, the membrane surrounding the ovum becomes _____ through a process termed the _____.

3. With the fusion of the male and female_____, the _____ number of chromosomes is restored. The new cell is called a _____. Within _____ days, a 16-cell ball called the _____ is formed. A cavity develops within this ball of cells, creating the _____ which is _____ into the endometrium _____ days after conception. The endometrium is now called the _____. Fingerlike projections called _____ develop from the _____. These projections tap into maternal blood vessels in the decidua _____.

4. Each of the following structures plays a critical role in fetal growth and development. List the functions of each of the structures listed below:

   Yolk sac

   Amniotic membranes and fluid

   Umbilical cord

Placenta

5. Fetal circulation differs from neonatal circulation. Describe the location and purpose for each of the following fetal circulatory structures:

Ductus venosus

Ductus arteriosus

Foramen ovale

True or False

Circle "T" if true or "F" if false for each of the following statements. Correct the false statements.

T   F   6. All normal human somatic cells contain 46 chromosomes.

T   F   7. Hemophilia and color blindness are examples of sex chromosome abnormalities caused by mutation during gametogenesis in either parent.

T   F   8. Neural tube defects, cleft lip and palate, pyloric stenosis, and congenital heart disease result from a combination of genetic and environmental factors.

T   F   9. In order for a recessive trait to be expressed in their offspring, both parents must contribute the abnormal gene.

T   F   10. In autosomal dominant inheritance, if one parent is affected by the disorder, there is a 100% chance of passing the abnormal gene to an offspring during each pregnancy.

T   F   11. Cystic fibrosis and phenylketonuria (PKU) are both inborn errors of metabolism and autosomal dominant inherited disorders.

T   F   12. The stage of the fetus lasts from 9 weeks gestation until the end of pregnancy, at about 40 weeks gestation.

T   F   13. The umbilical cord is composed of one vein, two arteries, Wharton's jelly, ligaments, and nerves.

T   F   14. Human chorionic gonadotrophin (hCG) is first detected in maternal blood 3 weeks after conception and begins to decrease at about 24 weeks gestation.

T   F   15. The corpus luteum produces estrogen and progesterone to maintain the pregnancy until the placenta is mature enough to take over as an endocrine gland.

T   F   16. The placenta functions as an effective barrier to substances such as viruses and drugs, thereby protecting the fetus from their potentially harmful effects.

T   F   17. Oligohydramnios often indicates fetal renal dysfunction.

T   F   18. Meconium, fetal waste products in the intestine of a fetus, may be passed into the amniotic fluid if fetal hypoxia occurs.

T   F   19. If a couple give birth to a child with an autosomal dominant disorder, there is a 50% reduction in risk that the next pregnancy will result in an affected child.

T   F   20. Fetal viability is first reached at 30 weeks gestation.

T   F   21. A human pregnancy reaches term by 40 weeks or 280 days.

T   F   22. The occurrence of multifetal pregnancies with three or more fetuses has steadily decreased as a result of increased exposure to teratogens.

23. Genetic counseling is rapidly becoming an important health-care service for families during the childbearing years.
    A. State the purposes for genetic counseling.

    B. Discuss each of the following steps in the process of genetic counseling.
       Estimation of risk

       Interpretation of risk

    C. Describe the nurse's role in genetic counseling.

24. Name the three primary germ layers and identify the tissues or organs that develop from each layer.

Primary germ layer	Tissue/organ formation

25. Identify five factors to include in a health history interview to determine a pregnant woman's risk for inheritable disorders.

26. Explain each of the following types of inheritance and give an example of each:
Unifactorial inheritance

Multifactorial inheritance

X-Linked inheritance

Critical Thinking Exercises

1. Imagine that you are a nurse-midwife working in partnership with an obstetrician. Formulate a response to each of the following concerns or questions directed to you from some of your prenatal patients:
   A. June (two months pregnant), Mary (five months pregnant), and Alice (seven months pregnant) each ask for a description of their fetus at the present time.
   June   **Mary**   **Alice**

   B. Jessica states that a friend told her that babies born after about 35 weeks have a better chance to survive because they can breathe easier. She asks if this is true.

   C. Beth, who is one month pregnant, states that she heard that women who are pregnant experience quickening. She wants to know what that could mean and if it hurts.

D. Susan, who is six months pregnant, states that she read in a magazine that a fetus can actually hear and see. She feels that this is totally unbelievable!

E. Alexa is two months pregnant. She asks how the sex of her baby was determined and if a sonogram could tell if she was having a boy or a girl.

F. Karen is pregnant for the first time. She reveals that she has a history of twins in her family. She wants to know what causes twin pregnancies to occur and what the difference is between identical and fraternal twins.

2. Mr. and Mrs. Goldberg are newly married and are planning for pregnancy. They express to the nurse their concern that Mrs. Goldberg has a history of Tay-Sachs disease in her family. Mr. Goldberg has never investigated his family history.
   A. Describe the process the nurse should follow in assisting the Goldbergs to determine their genetic risk.

   B. Both Mr. and Mrs. Goldberg are found to be carriers of the disorder. Describe the risk they have for giving birth to a child who is normal, is a carrier, or is affected by the disorder.

   C. Discuss the decision-making process that should be followed with couples like Mr. and Mrs. Goldberg who could give birth to a child with a genetic disorder.

Crossword Puzzle

Genetics, Conception, and Fetal Development

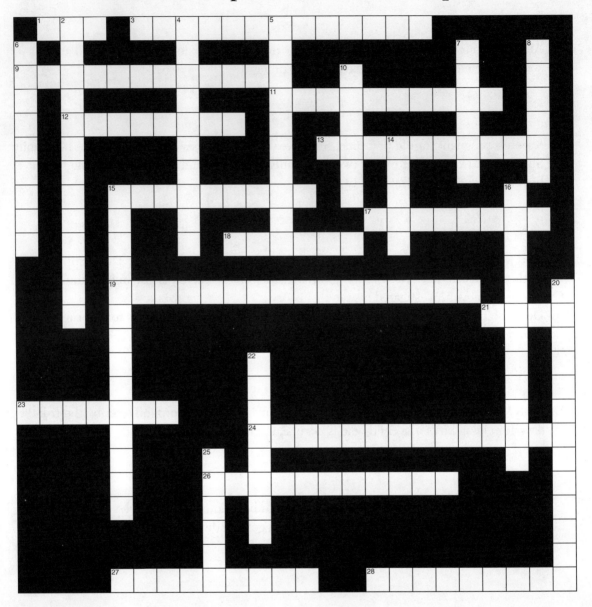

Across

1. Protein hormone found in maternal serum and urine after conception.

3. Structure that attaches the embryo/fetus to the placenta.

9. Attachment process whereby the blastocyst burrows into the endometrium beneath it.

11. Threadlike strands formed of DNA.

12. The _____ membranes enclose the embryo/fetus and the fluid that surrounds it.

13. Phospholipid formed by cells in the alveoli to facilitate respiration after birth.

15. Two zygotes are formed resulting in fraternal or _____ twins.

17. A spontaneous and permanent change in the normal gene structure.

18. The copy of genetic material in humans.

19. Opening between the fetal pulmonary artery and aorta.

21. A small segment of DNA found on chromosomes.

23. Process of cell division used to produce ova and sperm, each of which contain 23 chromosomes.

24. Finger-like projections that develop out of the trophoblast and extend into the endometrium.

26. One zygote divides resulting in identical or _____ twins.

27. A pictorial analysis of the number, form, and size of an individual's chromosomes.

28. Environmental substance or exposure that cause adverse effects on fetal development.

Down

2. Head-to-rump direction of growth and development.

4. Term used for the developing embryo when a cavity forms within the mass of cells.

5. Union of a single egg and sperm, marking the beginning of a pregnancy.

6. Capability of the fetus to survive outside the uterus.

7. The male and female germ cells.

8. Single cell resulting from the process of fertilization.

10. Solid ball of 16 cells formed within three days of fertilization.

14. Term used for the developing baby from 9 weeks gestation to end of pregnancy.

15. Portion of the endometrium directly under the blastocyst at implantation; it is where the chorionic villi tap into the maternal blood vessels.

16. Opening or shunt between the right and the left atria of the fetal heart.

20. Process whereby sperm penetrates ovum.

22. Structure formed of 15 to 20 cotyledons through which the chorionic villi branch out.

25. The developing baby from day 15 until about 8 weeks from conception.

CHAPTER 9

Anatomy and Physiology of Pregnancy

Chapter Review Activities

Fill in the Blanks

Insert the term that corresponds to each of the following definitions.

1. _____ Pregnancy.
2. _____ The number of pregnancies in which the fetus or fetuses have reached viability, not the number of fetuses (e.g., twins) born. Whether the fetus is born alive or is stillborn (fetus who shows no signs of life at birth) after viability is reached has no effect on the numerical designation.
3. _____ A woman who is pregnant.
4. _____ A woman who has never been pregnant.
5. _____ A woman who has not completed a pregnancy with a fetus or fetuses who have reached the stage of fetal viability.
6. _____ A woman who is pregnant for the first time.
7. _____ A woman who has completed one pregnancy with a fetus or fetuses who have reached the stage of fetal viability.
8. _____ A woman who has had two or more pregnancies.
9. _____ A woman who has completed two or more pregnancies to the stage of fetal viability.
10. _____ Capacity to live outside the uterus, about 22 to 24 weeks since the last menstrual period, or greater than 500 g.
11. _____ Born after 20 weeks of gestation but before completion of 37 weeks of gestation.
12. _____ Born between the beginning of 38 weeks of gestation and the end of 42 weeks of gestation.
13. _____ Born after 42 weeks of gestation.
14. _____ Its presence in urine or serum results in a positive pregnancy test result.

Matching

Match the assessment finding in Column I with the appropriate descriptive term in Column II.

COLUMN I

_____ 15. Menstrual bleeding no longer occurs.

_____ 16. Fundal height decreased, fetal head in pelvic inlet

_____ 17. Cervix and vagina violet-bluish in color

_____ 18. Swelling of ankles and feet

_____ 19. Cervical tip softened

_____ 20. Increased hair growth on face and abdomen

_____ 21. Fetal head rebounds with gentle, upward tapping through the vagina

_____ 22. White mucoid vaginal discharge with faint, musty odor

_____ 23. Plug of mucus fills endocervical canal

_____ 24. Pink stretch marks on breasts and abdomen

_____ 25. Thick, creamy fluid expressed from nipples

_____ 26. Cheeks, nose, and forehead blotchy, hyperpigmented

_____ 27. Pigmented line extending up abdominal midline

_____ 28. Varicosities around the anus

_____ 29. Heartburn experienced after supper

_____ 30. Lumbosacral curve increased

_____ 31. Spotting following cervical palpation or intercourse

_____ 32. Hematocrit decreased from 40% to 36%

_____ 33. Vascular spiders on neck and thorax

_____ 34. Pinkish red, mottled palms

_____ 35. Abdominal wall muscles separated

COLUMN II

A. Colostrum

B. Operculum

C. Amenorrhea

D. Telangiectasis (angioma)

E. Pyrosis

F. Friability

G. Striae gravidarum

H. Physiologic anemia

I. Linea nigra

J. Ballottement

K. Chadwick's sign

L. Diastasis recti abdominis

M. Lordosis

N. Leukorrhea

O. Chloasma (mask of pregnancy)

P. Lightening

Q. Hemorrhoids

R. Palmar erythema

S. Goodell's sign

T. Physiologic edema

U. Hirsutism

36. Complete the following table related to the three categories of signs and symptoms of pregnancy by filling in the blanks and listing the appropriate signs and symptoms for each category.

_____, those changes felt by the woman.	_____, those changes observed by an examiner.	_____, those signs attributed only to the presence of the fetus.

37. Describe the obstetric history for each of the following women, using the 4-digit and 5-digit system.

A. Nancy is pregnant. Her first pregnancy resulted in a stillbirth at 36 weeks gestation and her second pregnancy resulted in the birth of her daughter at 42 weeks gestation.

4-digit

5-digit

B. Marsha is 6 weeks pregnant. Her previous pregnancies resulted in the live birth of a daughter at 40 weeks gestation, the live birth of a son at 38 weeks gestation, and a spontaneous abortion at 10 weeks gestation.

4-digit

5-digit

C. Linda is experiencing her fourth pregnancy. Her first pregnancy ended in a spontaneous abortion at 12 weeks, the second resulted in the live birth of twin boys at 32 weeks, and the third resulted in the live birth of a daughter at 39 weeks.

4-digit

5-digit

True or False

Circle "T" if true or "F" if false for each of the following statements. Correct the false statements.

T   F   38. Pregnancy tests are based on the presence of human chorionic gonadotrophin (hCG) in a woman's urine or serum.

T   F   39. Urine pregnancy tests are more accurate and sensitive than serum pregnancy tests and can provide earlier results.

T   F   40. Drugs such as antibiotics can contribute to a false pregnancy test result.

T   F   41. Fetal movements palpated by an examiner are an example of a positive sign of pregnancy.

T   F   42. The uterine fundus should be above the level of the symphysis pubis by the eighth week of gestation.

T   F   43. Cervical mucus present during pregnancy does not exhibit ferning as a result of the influence of progesterone.

T   F   44. During pregnancy, the pH of vaginal secretions decreases, thereby increasing the woman's risk for viral genital tract infections.

T   F   45. Lactation does not occur during pregnancy as a result of the inhibiting effect of high estrogen and progesterone levels.

T   F   46. Physiologic anemia is diagnosed in a pregnant woman when the hemoglobin value falls to 10 gm/dl or less or if the hematocrit value falls to 35% or less.

T   F   47. A woman is at greater risk for the development of thrombophlebitis during pregnancy and the postpartum period as a result of increases in certain clotting factors and depression of fibrinolytic activity.

T   F   48. Pregnancy is a state of respiratory alkalosis compensated by a mild metabolic acidosis.

T   F   49. A supine position with head elevated is the best maternal position to facilitate renal perfusion.

T   F   50. A proteinuria of 1+ or less is acceptable during pregnancy.

T   F   51. Hypercalcemia is common during pregnancy and can result in leg cramps and tetany.

T   F   52. Perspiration increases during pregnancy as a result of increased peripheral circulation and increased sweat gland activity.

T   F   53. Carpal tunnel syndrome, especially in the dominant hand, can occur during the third trimester of pregnancy as a result of edema, which compresses the median nerve beneath the carpal ligament in the wrist.

T   F   54. Increased triglyceride and estrogen levels may account for the tendency to develop gallstones during pregnancy.

T   F   55. During the first half of pregnancy, maternal glucose supplies are preserved for the fetus by decreasing the pregnant woman's ability to utilize her own insulin.

56. When the nurse assesses the pregnant woman, baseline vital sign values will change as she progresses through her pregnancy.
    A. Describe how each of the following would change:
    Blood pressure

    Heart rate and patterns

    Respiratory rate and patterns

    Body temperature

57. Calculate the mean arterial pressure (MAP) for each of the following blood pressure readings:

   120/76

   114/64

   110/80

   150/90

58. Specify the value changes that occur in the following laboratory tests as a result of expected physiologic adaptations to pregnancy:

   CBC: hematocrit, hemoglobin, white blood cell count

   Clotting activity

   Acid-base balance

   Urinalysis

59. Describe the expected adaptations in elimination that occur during pregnancy. Include in your answer the basis for the changes that occur.

   Renal   **Bowel**

60. Explain how and why the levels of each of the following substances change during pregnancy.
    A. Parathyroid hormone

    B. Insulin

    C. Estrogen

    D. Progesterone

    E. Thyroid hormones

    F. Human chorionic gonadotrophin (hCG)

Crossword Puzzle

The Pregnant Woman and Family

Complete this puzzle after reading and studying Chapters 9, 10, and 11.

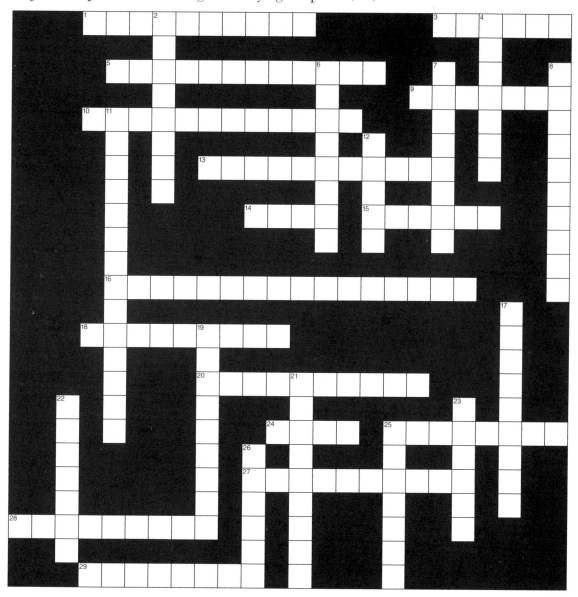

Across

1. Maternal perception of fetal movement.

3. Softening and compressibility of the lower uterine segment is termed _____ sign.

5. Uterine contractions felt through the abdominal wall after the fourth month of pregnancy are referred to as _____ sign.

9. Specific culturally based paternal behaviors associated with pregnancy.

10. Sound produced by fetal blood flowing through the umbilical cord; synchronous with the fetal heart rate.

13. Experiencing conflicting feelings about being pregnant.

14. Word used to describe an infant born between the beginning of the 38th week of gestation and the end of the 42nd week of gestation.

15. Red, raised nodule on the gums that bleeds easily.

16. Stretch marks.

18. Hypertrophied sebaceous glands in the areola are called Montgomery's _____.

20. Fundal height drops as the fetus begins to descend and engage in the pelvis.

24. Practice of consuming nonfood substances or excessive amounts of foodstuffs low in nutritional value.

25. Excessive salivation.

27. Cessation of menstruation.

28. Mucous plug that fills the endocervical canal.

29. Rapid and unpredictable changes in mood are termed emotional _____.

Down

2. Urge to eat specific types of foods such as ice cream, pickles, or pizza.

4. A woman who is pregnant.

6. Mask of pregnancy.

7. Softening of the cervical tip is referred to as _____ sign.

8. White or slightly gray mucoid vaginal discharge with a faint musty odor.

11. Rushing or blowing sound of maternal blood flowing though uterine arteries; synchronous with the maternal heart beat.

12. Pelvic floor exercises to strengthen the muscles around the reproductive organs and improve muscle tone.

17. Increased vascularity of vagina and cervix resulting in a violet-bluish color is referred to as _____ sign.

19. Creamy white to yellowish premilk fluid.

21. One of the three 3-month periods composing the prenatal period.

22. Formula used to estimate the date of birth is called _____ rule.

23. Psychoprophylactic method of childbirth.

25. Heartburn or "acid indigestion"

26. Number of pregnancies in which the fetus or fetuses have reached viability.

Critical Thinking Exercises

1. Describe your response to each of the following patient concerns and questions.
   A. Tina is 14 weeks pregnant. She calls the prenatal clinic to report that she noticed slight, painless spotting this morning. She reveals that she did have intercourse with her partner the night before.

   B. Lisa suspects she is pregnant since her menstrual period is already three weeks late. She asks her friend, who is a nurse, how to use the pregnancy test that she just bought so that she obtains the best results.

   C. Joan is 3 months pregnant. She tells you that she is worried because a friend told her that vaginal and bladder infections are more common during pregnancy. She wants to know if this could be true and if so why.

   D. Tammy, who is 20 weeks pregnant, tells you that she has noted some "problems" with her breasts: there are "little pimples" near her nipples and her breasts feel "lumpy and bumpy" and "leak a little" when she does a breast self-examination.

E. Tamara is concerned since she read in a book about pregnancy that a pregnant woman's position could affect her circulation, especially to the baby. She asks what positions are good for her circulation now that she is pregnant.

F. Beth, a pregnant woman, calls to tell you she had a nosebleed this morning and has noticed occasional feelings of fullness in her ears. She asks if these occurrences are anything to worry about.

G. Karen is 7 months pregnant and works full time as a secretary. She asks you if she should take a "water pill" that a friend gave her since she has noticed that her ankles "swell up" at the end of the day.

H. Jan is in her third trimester of pregnancy. She tells you that her posture seems to have changed and that she occasionally experiences low back pain.

I. Monica, who is 36 weeks pregnant with her first baby, calls the clinic stating that she knows the baby is coming since she felt some uterine contractions before getting out of bed in the morning. Monica confirms that they seem to have decreased in intensity and frequency since she has gotten out of bed and walked around.

J. Nina is a primigravida who is at 32 weeks gestation. When she comes for a prenatal visit she reports that she has been experiencing occasional periods of shortness of breath during the day and sometimes has to use an extra pillow to sleep comfortably. Nina expresses concern that she is developing a breathing problem.

2. Accurate blood pressure readings are critical, if significant changes in the cardiovascular system are to be detected as a woman adapts to pregnancy during the prenatal period. Write a protocol for blood pressure assessment that can be used by nurses working in a prenatal clinic to ensure accuracy of the results obtained during blood pressure assessment.

CHAPTER 10

Nursing Care During Pregnancy

Chapter Review Activities

Fill in the Blanks

Insert the term that corresponds to each of the following descriptions.

1. Pregnancy can be diagnosed by assessing a woman for the presence of specific signs and symptoms associated with pregnancy. _____ indicators of pregnancy can be caused by conditions other than gestation and are not reliable for diagnosis. _____ indicators of pregnancy are those observed by the health-care provider. _____ indicators of pregnancy verify that a woman is pregnant.

2. _____ rule is used to determine the _____ by subtracting _____ from and adding _____ to the first day of the _____. Pregnancy is divided into three 3-month periods called _____. The duration of most pregnancies is 38 to 40 weeks.

3. _____ can occur when a woman is placed in the lithotomy position as a result of the compression of the vena cava and aorta by the weight of the abdominal contents, including the uterus. Signs and symptoms that this has occurred would include _____, _____, _____, _____, _____, and _____.

4. A variety of assessment methods are used to evaluate the progress of pregnancy. _____ is measured beginning in the second trimester as one indicator of the progress of fetal growth. The _____ test determines whether the nipple is everted or inverted, by placing thumb and forefinger on the areola and pressing inward gently.

5. The well being of the fetus or _____ is assessed by evaluating _____, _____, and _____. The fetal _____ is estimated after determining the duration of pregnancy and the estimated date of birth.

6. Maternal adaptation during pregnancy includes mastery of certain _____ tasks that include _____, _____, _____, _____, and _____.

7. As a pregnant woman establishes a relationship with her fetus, she progresses through three phases. In phase one, she accepts the _____ and needs to be able to state _____. In phase two, the woman accepts the _____ and a _____. She can now say _____. Finally, in phase three, the woman prepares realistically for _____ and _____. She expresses the thought _____.

8. The _____ phase is the early period of paternal adaptation when the father accepts the biologic fact of pregnancy. During the _____ phase the father adjusts to the reality of the pregnancy. The father becomes actively involved in the pregnancy and the relationship with his child during the _____ phase.

9. The _____ is a tool used by parents to communicate the childbirth options they have chosen to their health care providers.

10. Certain cultural practices are expected by women of all cultures to ensure a good outcome to their pregnancy. Cultural _____ are directives that tell a woman what to do during pregnancy. Cultural _____ are directives that tell a woman what not to do during pregnancy; they establish _____ .

11. The multiple marker or triple screen test is used to detect _____ . It is done between _____ weeks gestation and measures _____ , _____ , and _____ .

12. Pregnancy often is the beginning of or escalation in violence.
    A. State the harmful effects of battering during pregnancy.

    B. List the target body parts for battering.

    C. Identify the difficulties pregnant women may report that can assist the nurse to determine that battering is taking place.

Matching

Match the description in Column I with the appropriate childbirth option in Column II.

COLUMN I

_____ 13. Place of birth that is outside the hospital and is staffed by physicians who have privileges at the local hospital and by certified nurse-midwives who are prepared to attend to low-risk pregnant women.

_____ 14. Hospital room designed for the childbirth process and the early recovery period. Women are then transferred to the postpartum unit.

_____ 15. Place of birth that may be physically separate from or part of the traditional obstetric department of a hospital. Homelike accommodations are typical of this place of birth.

_____ 16. Birth that takes place in the expectant family's own living environment.

_____ 17. Hospital room designed to accommodate a laboring woman and her family from admission to discharge during the postpartum period. No transfer to a separate postpartum unit is required.

COLUMN II

A. Alternative birth center

B. Free-standing birth center

C. Home birth

D. LDR room

E. LDRP room

18. Calculate the expected date of birth (EDB) for each of the following pregnant women using Nägele's rule.
    A. Diane's last menses began on May 5, 1998 and the last day occurred on May 10, 1998.

    B. Sara had intercourse on February 21, 1997. She has not had a menstrual period since the one that began on January 14, 1997 and ended 5 days later.

    C. Beth's last period began on July 4, 1998 and ended on July 10, 1998. Dawn noted that her basal body temperature (BBT) began to rise on July 28, 1998.

19. Cultural beliefs and practices are important influencing factors during the prenatal period.
    A. Describe how cultural beliefs can affect a woman's participation in prenatal care as it is defined by the Western Biomedical Model of Care.

    B. Identify one **prescription** and one **proscription** for each of the following areas:
       Emotional responses

       Clothing

       Physical activity and rest

       Sexual activity

Dietary practices

20. Complete the following table by identifying data to be collected for each component of maternal assessment during the initial visit and follow-up visits during pregnancy.

Component	Initial visit	Follow-up visits
Interview and history		
Physical examination		
Laboratory and diagnostic testing		

21. Identify and describe each component of fetal assessment.

22. List the signs of potential complications (warning signs) for each trimester of pregnancy. Indicate possible cause(s) for each sign listed.

   First trimester   **Second/third trimester**

23. Describe the approach a nurse should take when discussing potential complications with a pregnant woman and her family.

True or False

Circle "T" if true or "F" if false for each of the following statements. Correct the false statements.

T   F   24. Weight-bearing exercises such as jogging and running should be avoided during pregnancy.

T   F   25. Elevation of maternal pulse above 100 beats/minute during exercise should be decreased since it can adversely affect uteroplacental perfusion.

T   F   26. The use of a condom is necessary during pregnancy if the woman is at risk for a sexually transmitted disease.

T   F   27. Intercourse is safe during a normal pregnancy as long as it is not uncomfortable.

T   F   28. Exposure to second-hand smoke is associated with fetal growth restriction and an increase in perinatal and infant morbidity and mortality.

T   F   29. It is not necessary to screen pregnant women for human immunodeficiency virus (HIV) since there is no effective measure to reduce transmission to the fetus.

T   F   30. A woman should be scheduled for prenatal visits once a month until the thirty-sixth week of pregnancy.

T   F   31. A one-hour glucose tolerance test is performed on all pregnant women at 28 weeks gestation to screen for the presence of gestational diabetes.

T   F   32. A rise in systolic blood pressure of 15 mm Hg or more and/or in diastolic blood pressure of 10 mm Hg or more above baseline should be viewed as an indicator of risk for pregnancy-induced hypertension.

T   F   33. The blood pressure reaches its lowest point during the second trimester (midpregnancy) and then returns to baseline by the end of the third trimester.

T   F   34. During the second and third trimesters (weeks 18 to 30) the height of the fundus in inches is approximately the same as the weeks gestation if the woman's bladder is full.

T   F   35. Quickening usually occurs between weeks 16 to 20 of gestation.

T   F   36. A woman should avoid tub bathing and shower instead once she reaches the midpoint of her pregnancy.

T   F   37. The side-lying position promotes uterine perfusion and fetoplacental oxygenation.

T   F   38. Once the uterus enlarges, the pregnant woman should use only the lap belt and avoid using a shoulder harness in an automobile.

T   F   39. A woman with inverted nipples should perform nipple rolling and tugging exercises during the third trimester to break adhesions.

T   F   40. Hepatitis B vaccination is contraindicated during pregnancy.

T   F   41. A sign of preterm labor would be uterine contractions every 10 minutes or more often (6 or more per hour) for one hour.

T   F   42. Breast shells can be used by women with inverted or flat nipples to help the nipples evert or become erect thereby facilitating latch on of the newborn once breastfeeding begins after birth.

T   F   43. Women who are positive for hepatitis B should not breastfeed.

T   F   44. Women often react to the confirmation of pregnancy with mixed feelings or ambivalence.

T   F   45. Emotional lability (mood swings) may be related to profound hormonal changes that are part of the maternal response to pregnancy.

T   F   46. Children typically respond to their mother's pregnancy in terms of their age and dependency needs.

47. Create a protocol for fundal measurement that will facilitate accuracy.

48. Identify four factors that can be used to estimate the gestational age of the fetus.

49. Describe three principles of body mechanics that pregnant woman should be taught to prevent injury.

50. Identify five safety guidelines that you would include in a pamphlet that addresses prevention of accidental injury during pregnancy. Include the rationale for each guideline identified.

51. During the third trimester, parents often make a decision concerning the method they will use to feed their newborn. List the contraindications for breastfeeding.

Critical Thinking Exercises

1. A health-history interview of the pregnant woman by the nurse is included as part of the initial prenatal visit.
   A. State the purpose of the health-history interview.

   B. List the components that should be included in the prenatal health history.

C. Write two questions for each component identified. Questions should be clear, concise, and understandable. Most of the questions should be open ended to elicit the most complete response from the patient.

2. Imagine that you are a nurse working in a prenatal clinic. You have been assigned to be the primary nurse for Martha, an 18-year-old, who has come to the clinic for confirmation of pregnancy. She tells you that she knows she is pregnant because she has already missed three periods, and a home pregnancy test that she did last week was positive. Martha states that she has had very little contact with the health-care system, and the only reason she came today is because her boyfriend insisted that she "make sure" she is really pregnant. Describe the approach that you would take regarding data collection and nursing intervention appropriate for this woman.

3. Terry is a primigravida in her first trimester of pregnancy. She is accompanied by her husband Tim to her second prenatal visit. Answer each of the following questions asked by Terry and Tim:
   A. "At the last visit I was told that my estimated date of birth is December 25! Can I really count on my baby being born on Christmas Day?"

   B. "Before I became pregnant my friend told me I should be doing Kegel exercises. I was too embarrassed to ask her about them. What are they and is it safe for me to do them while I am pregnant?"

   C. "What effect will pregnancy have on our sex life? We are willing to abstain during pregnancy if we have to, to keep our baby safe."

D. "This morning sickness I am experiencing is driving my crazy. I become nauseous in the morning and again late in the afternoon. Occasionally I vomit or have the dry heaves. Will this last for my entire pregnancy? Is there anything I can do to feel better?"

4. Tara is 2 months pregnant. She tells the nurse at the prenatal clinic that she is used to being active and exercises everyday. Now that she is pregnant she wonders if she should reduce or stop her exercise routine. Discuss the nurse's response to Tara.

5. Write one nursing diagnosis for each of the following situations. State one expected outcome and list appropriate nursing measures for the nursing diagnosis you identified.
   A. Beth is 6 weeks pregnant. During the health-history interview, she tells you that she has limited her intake of fluids and tries to hold her urine as long as she can because "I just hate having to go to the bathroom so frequently."
   Nursing diagnosis   **Expected outcome**   **Nursing measures**

   B. Doris, who is 23 weeks pregnant, tells you that she is beginning to experience more frequent lower back pain. You note that when she walked into the examining room her posture exhibited a moderate degree of lordosis and neck flexion. She was wearing shoes with 2-inch narrow heels.
   Nursing diagnosis   **Expected outcome**   **Nursing measures**

   C. Lisa, a primigravida at 32 weeks gestation, comes for a prenatal visit accompanied by her partner, the father of the baby. They both express anxiety about the impending birth of the baby and how they will handle the experience of labor. Lisa is especially concerned about how she will survive the pain, and her partner is primarily concerned about how he will help Lisa cope with labor and make sure she and the baby are safe.
   Nursing diagnosis   **Expected outcome**   **Nursing measures**

6. Molly and Mitch ask the nurse about a birth plan, stating that "our friends had one and they say it helped them to have a satisfying birthing experience."
   A. Describe a birth plan.

   B. State the purpose of a birth plan.

   C. Describe the approach the nurse should take in helping Molly and Mitch formulate a birth plan that is right for them.

7. Jane is a primigravida in her second trimester of pregnancy. Answer each of the following questions asked by Jane during a prenatal visit.
   A. "Why do you measure my abdomen every time I come in for a check up?"

   B. How can you tell if my baby is doing okay?"

   C. "I am going to start changing the way that I dress now that I am beginning to show. Do you have any suggestions I could follow, especially since I have a limited amount of money to spend?"

   D. "What can I do about gas and constipation? I never had much of a problem before I was pregnant."

E. "Since yesterday I have started to feel itchy all over. Do you think I am coming down with some sort of infection?"

F. "I will be flying to Chicago to visit my father in one month. Is airline travel safe for me when I am 5 months pregnant?"

8. While a nurse is measuring a pregnant woman's fundus, the woman becomes pale and diaphoretic. The woman, who is at 23 weeks gestation, states that she feels dizzy and light-headed.
   A. State the most likely explanation for the assessment findings exhibited by this woman.

   B. Describe the nurse's immediate action.

9. Kelly is a primigravida in her third trimester of pregnancy. Answer each of the following questions asked by Kelly during a prenatal visit.
   A. "My husband and I have decided to breastfeed our baby but friends told me it is very difficult if my nipples do not come out. Is there any way I can tell now if my nipples are okay for breastfeeding?"

   B. "My ankles are swollen by the time I get home from work late in the afternoon (Kelly teaches second grade). I have been trying to drink about 3 liters of fluid every day. Should I reduce the amount of liquid I am drinking or ask my doctor for a water pill?"

C. "I woke up last night with a terrible cramp in my leg. It finally went away but my husband and I just did not know what to do. What if this happens again tonight?"

10. Marge, a pregnant woman (2 - 0 - 0 - 1 - 0) beginning her third trimester, expresses concern about preterm birth. "I already had one miscarriage and my sister's baby died after being born too early."
    A. Indicate what the nurse can teach Marge about the signs of preterm labor.

    B. Describe the actions Marge should take if she experiences signs of preterm labor.

11. Carol is 4 months pregnant and beginning to "show." She asks the nurse what she should expect as a reaction from her 13-year-old daughter and 3-year-old son. Describe the response the nurse would make.

12. Your neighbor, Jane Smith, is in her second month of pregnancy. Knowing that you are a nurse, her husband Tom confides in you that he just cannot "figure Jane out. One minute she is happy and the next minute she is crying for no reason at all! I do not know how I will be able to cope with this for seven more months." Discuss how you would respond to his concern.

13. Jim's partner, Mary, is 5 months pregnant. He tells you that sometimes he feels "left out" of Mary's pregnancy and asks you if he is important to Mary as her partner and the father of the baby. Specify how you would answer his question.

14. Tony and Andrea are hoping to deliver their second baby at home. They have been receiving prenatal care from a certified nurse midwife who has experience with home birth. Their 5-year-old son and both sets of grandparents will be present for the birth. Discuss the preparation measures you would recommend to Tony and Andrea to ensure a safe and positive experience for everyone.

CHAPTER 11

Maternal and Fetal Nutrition

Chapter Review Activities

Fill in the Blanks

Insert the term that corresponds to each of the following descriptions.

1. Maternal malnutrition may impair fetal growth and development resulting in
_____. _____ is defined as a birth weight of 2,500 g (5½ pounds) or
less. Low-birth-weight (LBW) infants may be _____ and/or _____.
Poor weight gain early in pregnancy increases the risk for giving birth to a _____
infant, whereas inadequate gains during the last half of pregnancy increase the risk for
_____.

2. When individualizing the recommended daily allowances for pregnant and lactating
women, nurses need to consider variations in a pregnant woman's situation including
_____, _____, _____, _____, and _____.
_____ needs are met by carbohydrates, fats, and protein in the diet and should
be increased during the second and third trimesters _____ above prepregnancy
needs.

3. Women at greatest risk for inadequate protein intake would include _____,
_____, and _____.

4. Inadequate intake of iron can lead to the development of _____ during
pregnancy, a nutritional health problem that is more common among _____ and
_____ than among adult Caucasian women.

5. _____ is the inability to digest milk sugar because of the absence of the lactase
enzyme in the small intestine.

6. _____ is the practice of consuming nonfood substances such as _____
or _____ or excessive amounts of foodstuffs low in nutritional value such as
_____ or _____. _____ is the urge to consume specific types
of foods such as ice cream, pickles, and pizza.

7. Assessment of nutritional status begins with a diet history that should include
_____, _____, and _____. Physical examination includes
_____ measurements such as _____ and _____. Calculation
of the _____ is a method of evaluating the appropriateness of weight for height
and is used to guide a woman's weight gain during pregnancy.

8. Vegetarian diets can vary in terms of the foods allowed. Basic to all vegetarian diets are
_____, _____, _____, _____, _____,
and _____. A _____ diet includes fish, poultry, eggs, and dairy
products but does not allow beef or pork. _____ consume dairy products and
plant products. _____ or _____ consume only plant products.

9. _____ or heartburn is caused by reflux from the stomach into the esophagus.

10. Complete the following table by stating the importance of each of the following nutrients for healthy maternal adaptation to pregnancy and optimum fetal growth and development. Indicate the major food sources for each nutrient.

Nutrient	Importance for pregnancy	Common food sources
Protein		
Iron		
Calcium		
Zinc		
Fat-soluble vitamins (A, D)		
Water-soluble vitamins (folic acid, B_6, C)		

11. State five indicators of nutritional risk in pregnancy.

12. Identify two major guidelines that the nurse should follow when planning menus for a pregnant woman who is a strict vegetarian (vegan).

13. List four signs of good nutrition and four signs of inadequate nutrition.

14. Identify four nursing measures appropriate for each of the following nursing diagnoses:
    A. Alteration in nutrition: less than body requirements related to inadequate intake associated with moderate nausea and vomiting (morning sickness).

    B. Alteration in elimination, constipation, related to decreased intestinal motility associated with increased progesterone levels during pregnancy.

15. Determine the approximate body mass index (BMI) for each of the following pregnant women and indicate the recommended weight gain and pattern for each woman based on her calculated BMI.

Woman	BMI	Weight gain
June: 5 ft 3 in, 120 pounds		
Alice: 5 ft 6 in, 205 pounds		
Ann: 5 ft 5 in, 95 pounds		

True or False

Circle "T" if true or "F" if false for each of the following statements. Correct the false statements.

T   F   16. Good maternal nutrition before and during pregnancy is considered to be one of the most important preventive measures for LBW infants.

T   F   17. A series of 24-hour diet recalls is the best way to determine the appropriateness of a woman's Kcal intake.

T F 18. A woman whose BMI is 29 (over weight) should gain approximately 0.6 pound or 0.3 kg/per week during the second and third trimesters of pregnancy for a total of 15 to 25 pounds or 7 to 11.5 kg overall.

T F 19. Adolescents, especially those who are less than 2 to 3 years past menarche, are at greatest nutritional risk since their growth is in competition with that of the fetus for nutrients.

T F 20. A caloric increase of 600 kcal per day is recommended for pregnant women beginning in the first trimester.

T F 21. Ketonuria resulting from an inadequate intake of Kcals has been associated with preterm labor.

T F 22. Maternal anemia increases the risk for postpartum infection and poor wound healing.

T F 23. Pregnant women should avoid caffeine since research has indicated that caffeine can result in neonatal neurologic dysfunction.

T F 24. Women should begin taking an iron supplement starting at 12 weeks gestation.

T F 25. If moderate peripheral edema occurs during pregnancy, the woman's sodium intake should be reduced.

T F 26. Excessive intake of fat-soluble vitamins such as vitamin A during pregnancy can result in toxicity leading to congenital malformations of the fetus.

T F 27. Development of neural tube defects appears to be more common in the fetuses of pregnant women whose diet is low in vitamin B_6 and C.

T F 28. Dehydration can stimulate the onset of premature labor.

T F 29. Lactating women need to consume at least 2,500 kcal/day along with an adequate intake of calcium.

T F 30. Lactating women should be told that loss of the weight gained during pregnancy will begin after they stop breastfeeding.

T F 31. The most common nutrition-related laboratory test for a pregnant woman is a hematocrit and hemoglobin measurement.

T F 32. Smoking may impair the production of milk in lactating women.

T F 33. Caffeine intake can lead to a reduction in the concentration of iron in the milk of lactating women.

34. Identify three guidelines that should be followed to ensure adequate nutrition during lactation.

35. State four factors that contribute to the increase in nutrient needs during pregnancy.

Critical Thinking Exercises

1. Nutrition and weight gain are important areas of consideration for nurses who care for pregnant women. In addition, weight gain is often a source of stress and body image alteration for the pregnant woman. Discuss the approach you would use in each of the following situations.

A. Kelly (5 ft 8 in, 130 pounds) complains to you that her physician recommended a weight gain of approximately 30 pounds during her pregnancy. She states, " Babies only weigh about 7 pounds when they are born! Why do I have to gain much more than that?"

B. Kate (5 ft 4 in, 125 pounds) has just found out that she is pregnant. She states, "I am so glad to be pregnant. I love to eat, and now I can start eating for two. It will be great not to have to watch the scale or what I eat."

C. June tells you that she does not have to worry about her nutrient intake during her pregnancy. "I take plenty of vitamins—everything from A to Z!!"

D. Erin is 7 months pregnant. She asks you what she can do to relieve the heartburn she experiences after meals, especially dinner.

E. Sara (BMI = 28.7) is one month pregnant. She asks you for dietary guidance, including a weight reduction diet since she does not want to gain too much weight with this pregnancy.

F. Beth is 2 months pregnant. She states, "I have cut down on my water intake. I do get a little thirsty but it is worth it since I do not have to urinate so often."

G. Hedy is 2 months pregnant and has come for her second prenatal visit. During a discussion about nutrition needs during pregnancy she states, " I know I will not get enough calcium because I get sick when I drink milk."

H. Lara is 36 weeks pregnant. She states that she would like to breastfeed her baby but is concerned about getting back into shape and losing weight after the baby is born. "My friends told me that I will lose weight more slowly since I will not be able to start on a weight reduction diet as long as I am breastfeeding."

2. Yvonne's hemoglobin is 13 gm/dl and her hematocrit is 37% at the onset of her pregnancy. She asks the nurse if she will have to take iron during her pregnancy if she follows a good diet. "My friend took iron when she was pregnant and it made her sick to her stomach." Discuss the appropriate response by the nurse.

3. Gloria is an 18-year-old Native-American woman (5 ft 6 in, 98 pounds) who has just been diagnosed as 8 weeks pregnant. In her discussions with you at her first prenatal visit, she expresses a lack of knowledge regarding the nutritional requirements of pregnancy and wants to know what to eat since she wants to have a healthy baby.
   A. Outline the approach that you would use to help Gloria learn about and meet the nutritional requirements of her pregnancy.

   B. Plan a one-day menu that incorporates Gloria's nutritional needs and reflects the traditions of her culture.

Factors and Processes of Labor and Birth

Chapter Review Activities

Fill in the Blanks

Insert the term that corresponds to each of the following definitions.

1. Fontanels are _____ that are located where _____ in the fetal/neonatal skull _____.
2. Molding is the slight _____ of the _____ that occurs during childbirth.
3. Presentation refers to the _____ that enters the _____ first. The three main types are _____ (head first), _____ (buttocks first), and _____.
4. The presenting part is the part of the fetal body _____ during a _____. The three most common types are _____, _____, and _____.
5. The vertex presentation occurs when the fetal head is _____, making the _____ the fetal part first felt by the examining finger.
6. Fetal lie is the relationship of the _____. There are two types: longitudinal (vertical) when the _____ and transverse (horizontal) when the _____.
7. Attitude is the relationship of the _____. The most common type is one of _____.
8. The biparietal diameter is the _____ of the fetal skull. The suboccipitobregmatic diameter is the _____ of the fetal skull to enter the maternal pelvis when the fetal head is in full _____.
9. Fetal position refers to the relationship of the _____ to the _____.
10. Engagement occurs when the _____ of the presenting part has passed through the _____, reaching the level of the _____.
11. Station is the relationship of the _____ of the fetus to an imaginary line drawn between the _____. It is expressed in terms of _____ above or below the _____, thereby serving as a method of determining the progress of fetal _____.
12. Effacement refers to the _____ of the _____ during the _____ stage of labor. Degree of effacement is expressed in terms of _____.
13. Dilatation is the _____ or _____ of the _____ and the _____ that occurs once labor has begun. Degree of progress is expressed in _____ from _____.
14. Lightening occurs when the _____ into the _____ approximately _____ before term in the primigravida and at the _____ in the multiparous woman.

15. Bloody show is a _____ discharge representing the passage of the _____ as the cervix _____ in preparation for labor.

16. The mechanism of labor is the _____ of the _____, to facilitate passage through the _____. Also known as the seven _____ of labor, they include:

_____, _____, _____, _____, _____, _____, and _____.

17. _____ is a pushing method during the second stage of labor whereby the woman holds her breath and tightens her abdominal muscles. It is not recommended since it increases _____, reduces _____, and increases _____. As a result, fetal _____ can occur.

18. Identify and describe the five factors (the five P's) that affect the process of labor and birth. Include in your description the manner in which each factor affects the progress of childbirth.

19. List the events that occur during each of the four stages of labor.

20. Describe each of the cardinal movements of labor.

21. Label the following illustrations of the fetal skull and the maternal pelvis with the appropriate landmarks and diameters.

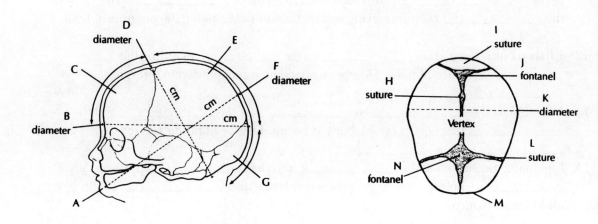

Fetal Skull

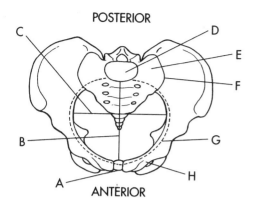

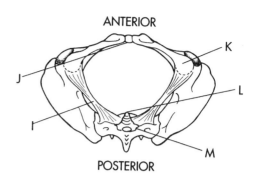

Pelvic Brim From Above

Pelvic Outlet From Above

Maternal Pelvis

22. Indicate the presentation, presenting part, position, lie, and attitude of the fetus for each of the following illustrations.

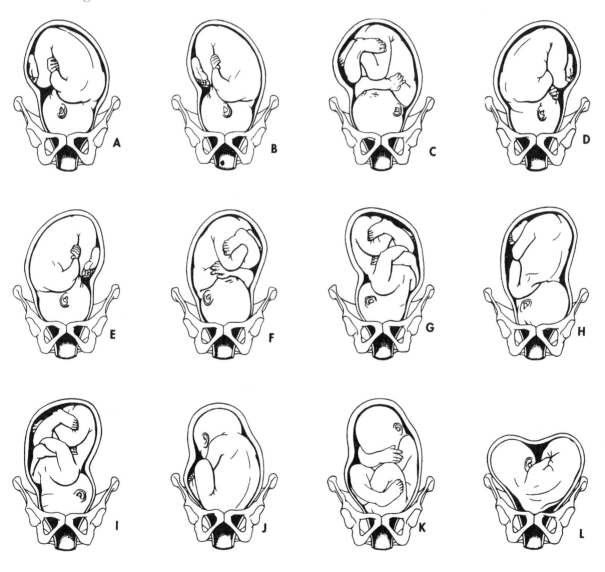

23. State the four factors that affect fetal circulation.

True or False

Circle "T" if true or "F" if false for each of the following statements. Correct the false statements.

T F 24. The most common fetal attitude is one of full extension of body parts.

T F 25. A longitudinal lie results in either a cephalic or a breech presentation.

T F 26. Fetal position is unlikely to change once labor begins.

T F 27. A woman must have a gynecoid pelvis to experience a spontaneous vaginal birth.

T F 28. Effacement usually precedes dilatation for a nulliparous woman but progresses simultaneously with dilatation for the multiparous woman.

T F 29. Women with a history of sexually transmitted disease may experience slowed or ineffective progress of cervical dilatation.

T F 30. The hands and knees position is most helpful when the fetal presentation is breech.

T F 31. Women often experience decreased dyspnea but increased urinary frequency after lightening occurs.

T F 32. The expected range of the fetal heart rate is 100 to 140 beats per minute for a full-term fetus.

T F 33. An increase in fetal pO_2 and arterial pH and a decrease in pCO_2 prepares the fetus for initiating respirations immediately after its birth.

T F 34. Because systolic blood pressure increases during a contraction by approximately 10 mm Hg, assessment of maternal blood pressure *between* contractions provides more accurate data.

T F 35. The white blood cell count increases to $35,000/mm^3$ or higher in response to the stress, tissue trauma, and increased activity level associated with childbirth.

T F 36. During labor, a woman should be encouraged to do leg exercises including pointing of toes to reduce the incidence of leg cramps.

T F 37. Endogenous endorphins secreted during labor raise a woman's pain threshold and enhance her ability to relax.

Crossword Puzzle

Labor and Birth

Complete this puzzle after reading Chapters 12, 13, 14, and 15.

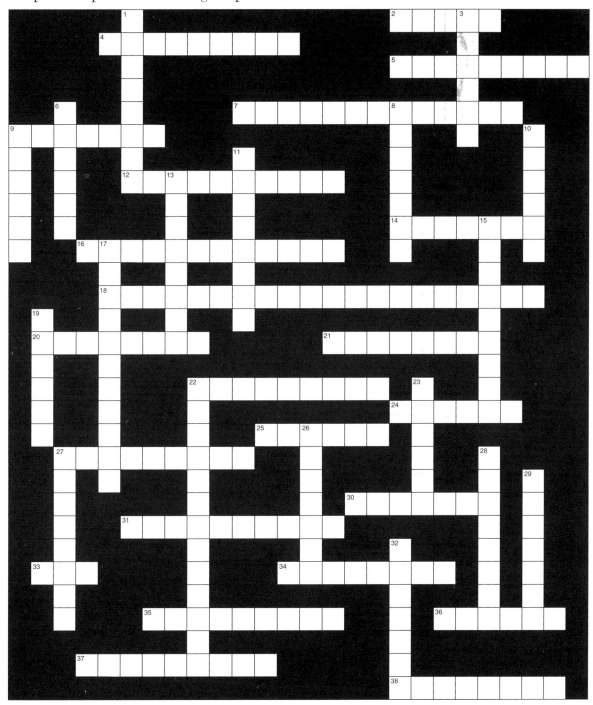

Across

2. The stage of labor during which the cervix widens and thins.

4. The cardinal movement of labor that facilitates the emergence of the fetal head.

5. The third stage of labor is the stage of _____ separation.

7. The level of the _____ is station zero. (2 words)

9. Overlapping of the fetal skull bones to facilitate its passage through the bony pelvis.

12. "Dropping" of the fetal presenting part into the true pelvis.

14. The reference point of a cephalic presentation when the head is fully flexed.

16. Term that refers to the part of the fetus that enters the pelvic inlet first.

18. The smallest anteroposterior diameter of the fetal skull.

20. Relationship of the fetal body parts to each other.

21. Softening of the cervix in preparation for labor's onset.

22. The _____ fontanel lies at the junction of the sagittal and lambdoidal sutures.

24. Another term used for the anterior fontanel.

25. When the cervix shortens and thins, it is said to _____.

27. The signs that a woman experiences before the onset of true labor are termed _____ labor.

30. Contractions of abdominal muscles and diaphragm are the secondary powers of labor.

31. For delivery to occur, the fetus must accommodate to this rigid passageway. (2 words)

33. Relationship of the fetal spine to the maternal spine.

34. Rotation maneuver to allow the fetal head to pass through the pelvic outlet is termed _____ rotation.

35. The time from the beginning of one uterine contraction to the beginning of the next.

36. When the cervical os widens or opens, it is said to _____.

37. Strength of a uterine contraction.

38. Length of a uterine contraction.

Down

1. The cardinal movement of labor that occurs as the fetal shoulders engage and descend through the pelvis is termed _____ rotation.

3. The stage of labor when the fetus is born.

6. Passage of cervical mucous plug before onset of labor is termed _____ show.

8. Measurement of fetal descent in relationship to the ischial spines.

9. Presenting part of a cephalic presentation when the fetal head is in extension.

10. The stage of recovery following delivery of the placenta.

11. Head-first presentation.

13. The most common type of pelvis for the female.

15. A labor curve or graph used to evaluate the progress of labor.

17. Realignment of the fetal head with its back and shoulders after the head is born.

19. Presenting part in a buttocks-first presentation.

22. Uterine contractions. (2 words)

23. Buttocks-first presentation.

26. Cardinal movement of labor that permits the smallest anteroposterior diameter of the fetal skull to pass through the pelvis.

27. Relationship of the presenting part to the four quadrants of the maternal pelvis.

28. Suture located between the two parietal bones of the fetal skull.

29. Downward progress of the presenting part through the pelvis.

32. When the biparietal diameter of the fetal head passes through the pelvic inlet, it is said to be _____.

Critical Thinking Exercises

1. As part of their care of the laboring woman, nurses perform vaginal examinations and interpret the results. State the meaning of each of the following vaginal examination findings.

Exam I	Exam II	Exam III	Exam IV
ROP	RMA	LST	OA
−1	0	+1	+3
50%	25%	75%	100%
3 cm	2 cm	6 cm	10 cm

2. Brooke is a primigravida at 36 weeks gestation. During a prenatal visit at 34 weeks gestation, she asks you the following questions regarding her approaching labor. Describe how you would respond to the following questions.

A. "What gets labor to start?"

B. "Are there things I should watch for that would tell me my labor is getting closer to starting?"

C. "How long can I expect my labor to last once it gets started?"

D. "My friend just had a baby and she told me the nurses kept helping her to change her position and even encouraged her to walk! Isn't that dangerous for the baby and painful for the mom?"

CHAPTER 13

Management of Discomfort

Chapter Review Activities

Fill in the Blanks

Insert the term that corresponds to childbirth pain for each of the following definitions.

1. _____ pain originates in the body organs during labor and birth. This type of pain results from _____ changes and uterine _____. It is located over the _____ of the abdomen and radiates to the _____ of the back and down the _____.

2. _____ pain originates in the muscles and bones. During labor and birth this type of pain is experienced as _____ pain that results from stretching of _____ to allow passage of the fetus and traction on the _____ and _____ during contractions.

3. _____ pain is felt in areas of the body other than the area of pain origin. During labor and birth this type of pain can be felt in the _____, _____, and _____.

4. The _____ Theory is based on the principle that certain nerve cell groupings within the spinal cord, brain stem, and cerebral cortex may have the ability to modulate the pain impulse through a blocking mechanism. According to this theory, pain sensations travel along sensory nerve pathways to the brain, and only a limited number of sensations or messages can travel through these nerve pathways at one time. Pain relief techniques based on this theory include _____ or _____, _____, _____, and _____.

5. _____ are endogenous opioids secreted by the pituitary gland that act on the central and peripheral nervous systems to reduce pain. It is thought that these opioid substances increase during pregnancy and birth in humans and may enhance the ability of the woman in labor to tolerate acute pain.

Insert the term that corresponds to nonpharmacologic techniques for management of discomfort for each of the following descriptions.

6. Three major childbirth preparation methods taught in the United States are _____, _____, and _____.

7. The basis of the _____ method, also know as natural childbirth, is to replace _____ with _____ and _____. This program includes information on _____, _____, _____, and _____. Classes include practice in three techniques: _____, _____, and _____. _____ respirations are recommended for most of labor, to be replaced by _____ toward the end of the first stage of labor.

8. The _____ method also known as the psychoprophylactic method is based on the belief that pain is a _____. This method conditions women to respond to mock uterine contractions with _____ and _____. _____ patterns vary according to the _____ and _____. Coping strategies also include _____ to keep nerve pathways occupied so they cannot respond to _____. Support in labor is provided by the woman's _____ or a specially trained labor attendant called a _____.

9. The _____ method is also know as husband-coached childbirth. This method emphasizes working in _____ using _____, _____, and _____. The technique stresses environmental factors such as _____, _____, and _____ to make childbirth a more natural experience.

10. Breathing techniques should be initiated when the laboring woman can no longer _____ or _____ through a contraction. _____ breathing is breathing at approximately _____ the woman's normal breathing rate. It is usually the first technique that is used in early labor.

11. As labor advances chest breathing is used with techniques becoming _____ in depth and increasing to about _____ the normal breathing rate.

12. A _____ should begin and end each breathing technique and contraction.

13. A breathing technique using a pattern of breaths and puffs in a ratio of 4:1, 6:1, or 8:1 is used to enhance concentration during the _____ phase of the first stage of labor. An undesirable effect of this type of breathing may be _____ or rapid deep respirations, which can result in _____ as exhibited by the symptoms of _____, _____, _____, and _____. It can be overcome by having the woman _____. This enables the woman to rebreathe _____.

14. _____ or light stroking of the abdomen or other body part in rhythm with breathing during contractions and _____ or steady pressure against the lower back especially during back labor are two examples of nonpharmacologic methods to relieve discomfort that are based on the _____ theory of pain.

15. _____ (i.e., whirlpool baths) uses the buoyancy of the warm water to provide support for tense muscles, relief from discomfort, and general body relaxation. It should not be initiated until the laboring woman is in the _____ phase of the first stage of labor. The temperature of the water must be maintained between _____ and _____ to prevent excessive elevation of the maternal _____ and a resulting increase in _____.

16. _____ uses two pairs of electrodes to provide continuous mild electrical currents that can be increased during a contraction. It may be effective because of a _____ effect which can stimulate the release of _____ in the woman's body and thereby alleviate discomfort.

17. Identify the factors that influence a laboring woman's pain response.

18. Explain the theoretic basis of such techniques as massage, stroking, music, and imagery in reducing the sensation of pain.

Matching

Match the description in Column I with the appropriate pharmacologic pain relief measure in Column II.

COLUMN I

_____ 19. Abolition of pain perception by interrupting nerve impulses going to the brain. Loss of sensation (partial or complete) and sometimes loss of consciousness occurs.

_____ 20. Method to repair a tear in the dura mater around the spinal cord as a result of spinal anesthesia.

_____ 21. Single-injection, subarachnoid anesthesia useful for pain control during birth but not for labor.

_____ 22. Systemic analgesic that provides analgesia without causing maternal or neonatal respiratory depression.

_____ 23. Provides rapid perineal anesthesia for performing and repairing an episiotomy

_____ 24. Anesthesia method used to relieve pain from lower uterine segment and cervix to upper third of vagina; has been associated with fetal complications related to rapid absorption of the drug.

_____ 25. Analgesic potentiators such as tranquilizers.

_____ 26. Drug that reverses effects of narcotics including neonatal narcosis (CNS depression of the newborn).

_____ 27. Medications such as narcotic analgesics that are administered IM or IV for pain relief during labor.

_____ 28. Alleviation of pain sensation or raising of the pain threshold without loss of consciousness.

_____ 29. Relief from pain of uterine contractions and birth by injecting a local anesthetic into the peridural space.

_____ 30. Anesthetic that eliminates vaginal, labial, and perineal pain making it useful for episiotomy, birth, and use of low forceps.

COLUMN II

A. Agonist-antagonist compounds
B. Anesthesia
C. Analgesia
D. Ataractics
E. Epidural block
F. Epidural blood patch
G. Local infiltration anesthesia
H. Spinal block
I. Narcotic antagonist
J. Paracervical block
K. Pudendal block
L. Systemic analgesia

31. Complete the following table by listing the effects, criteria/timing for use, and nursing management for each of the following commonly used nerve block anesthesias.

Anesthesia	Effects	Criteria/Timing	Management
Local Infiltration			
Pudendal block			
Spinal block			
Epidural block			

32. Systemic analgesics cross the placenta and affect the fetus.
    A. List three factors that influence the effect systemic analgesics have on the fetus.

    B. Describe the fetal effects of systemic analgesics.

33. Give one example for each of the following medication classifications and discuss how and why each example you cited is used during the childbirth process.
    Narcotic analgesic

Mixed narcotic agonist-antagonist compound

Analgesic potentiator

Narcotic antagonist

True or False

Circle "T" if true or "F" if false for each of the following statements. Correct the false statements.

T   F   34. Somatic pain occurs as a result of perineal stretching and pressure exerted by the presenting part on the pelvic organs and structures.

T   F   35. Pain threshold is highly variable among individuals and is affected by differences in terms of gender, social status, ethnicity, and culture.

T   F   36. A woman's perception of her birth experience as "good" or "bad" is influenced by the degree to which she believes she met the goals she set for herself in terms of coping with pain.

T   F   37. Water therapy can be used even if the laboring woman's membranes are ruptured.

T   F   38. A laboring woman should limit her time in a whirlpool bath to 30 minutes.

T   F   39. Effectiveness of acupressure is based on the gate control theory of pain and an increase in endorphin levels.

T   F   40. Sedatives such as barbiturates relieve anxiety and induce sleep in prodromal or early labor and active labor even in the presence of pain.

T   F   41. Intravenous administration of analgesics is preferred over intramuscular administration because the onset of the drug's effects is more reliable.

T   F   42. Narcan should be used cautiously if a woman has a substance dependency since signs and symptoms of maternal narcotic withdrawal can occur.

T   F   43. Before initiating epidural anesthesia a woman should be adequately hydrated using an IV of 5% glucose in water.

T   F   44. Epidural anesthesia is useful for labor and birth.

T   F   45. Keeping the woman in a flat position for at least 8 hours after birth is the most effective way to prevent postspinal headache.

T   F   46. The woman can be assisted into a sitting position for the induction of both spinal anesthesia and lumbar epidural blocks.

T   F   47. Maternal hypotension is a major adverse reaction to both spinal anesthesia and epidural blocks.

Critical Thinking Exercises

1. A nurse working with a group of expectant fathers is asked if there really is "a physical reason for all the pain women say they feel when they are in labor." Describe the response that this nurse should give.

2. Nurses working on childbirth units must be sensitive to their patients' pain experiences.
   A. Identify the physical signs and affective expressions of pain that nurses could expect to observe when a patient experiences pain.

   B. Describe specific measures nurses could use to alter the laboring woman's perception of pain.

3. On admission to the labor unit in the latent phase of labor, Mr. and Mrs. Timins (2 - 0 - 0 - 1 - 0) tell you that they are so glad they took Lamaze classes and did so much reading about child-birth. "We will not need any medication now that we know what to do. But most importantly our baby will be safe!" Describe how you would respond if you were their primary nurse for childbirth.

4. Imagine you are the nurse manager of a labor and birth unit. Major renovations are being planned for your unit and your input is required. You and your staff nurses believe that water therapy including the use of showers and jacuzzies is a beneficial nonpharmacologic method to relieve pain and discomfort and enhance the progress of labor. Discuss the rationale you would use to convince planners that installing a shower and spa into each birthing room is cost effective.

5. Tara has been in labor for 4 hours. Her blood pressure had been stable, averaging 130/80 when assessed between contractions, and the fetal heart rate (FHR) pattern consistently exhibited criteria of a reassuring pattern. A lumbar epidural block was initiated. Shortly afterward during assessment of maternal vital signs and FHR, Tara's blood pressure decreased to 102/60, and the FHR pattern began to exhibit a decrease in rate and variability.

   A. State what Tara is experiencing. Support your answer and explain the physiologic basis for what is happening to Tara.

   B. List the immediate nursing actions.

6. Moira, a primigravida, has elected a continuous epidural block as her pharmacologic method of choice during childbirth.

   A. Identify the assessment procedures that should be used to determine Moira's readiness for the initiation of the epidural block.

   B. Identify the preparation methods that should be implemented.

   C. Describe two positions you could help Moira assume for the induction of the epidural block.

   D. Outline the nursing care management interventions recommended while Moira is receiving the anesthesia to ensure her well-being and that of her fetus.

CHAPTER 14

Fetal Monitoring

Chapter Review Activities

Fill in the Blanks

Insert the term that corresponds to fetal monitoring for each of the following descriptions.

1. The goals of intrapartum fetal heart rate (FHR) monitoring are to identify and differentiate the _____ patterns from the _____ patterns that are indicative of fetal _____. _____ is characterized by a deficiency of oxygen in the arterial blood, whereas _____ is an inadequate supply of oxygen at the cellular level.

2. One method to asess fetal status is intermittent (periodic) _____ using a _____ or _____ to listen to the FHR.

3. _____ is the method used to continuously assess the FHR pattern. Two modes can be used to accomplish this method of assessment. External monitoring uses an _____ to assess the FHR pattern and a _____ to monitor the frequency and duration of contractions. Internal monitoring uses a _____ attached to the fetal presenting part to assess the FHR pattern and an _____ to monitor the frequency, duration, and intensity of contractions.

4. _____ (insufficient amniotic fluid) can lead to compression of the umbilical cord resulting in a _____ FHR pattern. _____ can be used to instill normal saline or Ringer's lactate solution into the uterine cavity via the intrauterine catheter for the purpose of adding fluid around the umbilical cord and thus prevent its compression during uterine contractions.

5. It is critical that a nurse working on a labor unit knows the factors associated with a reduction in fetal oxygen supply, the characteristics of a reassuring FHR pattern, and the characteristics of normal uterine activity. List the required information for each of the following:
   A. Factors associated with a reduction in fetal oxygen supply

   B. Characteristics of a reassuring FHR pattern

C. Characteristics of normal uterine activity

5. Identify the characteristics of nonreassuring FHR patterns.

Matching: FHR Patterns

Match the definition in Column I with the appropriate term from Column II.

COLUMN I

_____ 6. Average FHR range of 110-160 beats per minute (BPM) at term as assessed during the absence of uterine activity or between contractions.

_____ 7. Absence of the expected irregular fluctuations in the baseline FHR.

_____ 8. Persistent (longer than 10 minutes) baseline FHR below 110 BPM.

_____ 9. Visually apparent decrease in the FHR of 15 BPM or more below baseline that lasts more than 2 minutes but less than 10 minutes.

_____ 10. Changes from baseline patterns in FHR that occur with uterine contractions.

_____ 11. Persistent (longer than 10 minutes) baseline FHR above 160 BPM.

_____ 12. Expected irregular fluctuations of the baseline FHR of two or more cycles per minute as a result of the interaction of the sympathetic and parasympathetic nervous system.

_____ 13. FHR decrease shortly after onset of a contraction as a response to fetal head compression.

_____ 14. FHR decrease after the peak of the contraction in response to uteroplacental insufficiency.

_____ 15. FHR decrease any time during a contraction in response to umbilical cord compression.

_____ 16. Visually apparent abrupt increase in the FHR of 15 BPM or more above the baseline that lasts 15 seconds or more with return to baseline less than two minutes after onset.

_____ 17. Changes from baseline patterns in FHR that are not associated with uterine contraction.

COLUMN II

A. Acceleration
B. Early deceleration
C. Variability
D. Late deceleration
E. Variable deceleration
F. Tachycardia
G. Prolonged deceleration
H. Bradycardia
I. Baseline FHR
J. Undetected variability
K. Periodic changes
L. Episodic changes

18. Indicate the factors and data a nurse should use to determine if a FHR pattern is reassuring or nonreassuring.

Fill in the Blanks

In general, the recommended frequency of FHR assessment depends on the risk status of the mother and the stage of labor. Insert the appropriate time for each of the following assessment recommendations:

19. Obtain a _____-minute strip by electronic fetal monitoring (EFM) on all women admitted to the labor unit.

20. Low-risk patient (risk factors are absent during labor): auscultate FHR/assess tracing every _____ in the latent phase of the first stage of labor, every _____ in the active phase of the first stage of labor, and every _____ in the second stage of labor.

21. High-risk patient (risk factors are present during labor): auscultate FHR/assess tracing every _____ in the latent phase of the first stage of labor, every _____ in the active phase of the first stage of labor, and every _____ in the second stage of labor.

22. State the advantages and disadvantages of intermittent auscultation as a method of fetal assessment during childbirth.

23. Outline the guidelines that should be followed when monitoring the fetus using the intermittent auscultation method.

24. Indicate the legal responsibilities related to fetal monitoring for nurses who care for women during childbirth.

True or False

Circle "T" if true or "F" if false for each of the following statements. Correct the false statements.

T   F   25. A nonreassuring FHR pattern indicates that the fetus is compromised and is experiencing some degree of hypoxemia and/or hypoxia.

T   F   26. Auscultation should be performed during a uterine contraction and for at least 10 seconds after the end of the contraction.

T   F   27. FHR variability can temporarily decrease when the fetus is in a sleep state.

T   F   28. When external monitoring is used the ultrasound transducer and tocotransducer should be repositioned every four hours, and reddened skin areas gently massaged.

T   F   29. Maternal supine hypotensive syndrome reduces blood flow to the placenta resulting in fetal hypoxia as reflected in fetal bradycardia, decreased variability, and late decelerations.

T   F   30. Acceleration of the FHR associated with fetal movement is a reassuring sign.

T   F   31. Decelerations of the FHR may be benign or nonreassuring in terms of fetal well being.

T   F   32. Late deceleration patterns are characterized by a U or V shape with acceleration shoulders before and after the deceleration.

T   F   33. Early decelerations are nonreassuring patterns that typically occur in the second stage of labor with fetal descent and maternal bearing-down efforts.

T   F   34. The average intrauterine (intraamniotic) pressure range during a uterine contraction is 50 to 75 mm Hg.

T   F   35. The tocotransducer should be placed on the abdomen over the fundus.

T   F   36. The intrauterine pressure catheter (IUPC) is able to assess uterine contraction frequency, duration, and intensity.

T   F   37. Ritgen's maneuvers are used to determine the correct placement of the ultrasound transducer.

T   F   38. Late deceleration patterns of any magnitude are considered to be nonreassuring FHR patterns.

39. List the emergency measures that a nurse should implement when nonreassuring FHR patterns are identified.

40. State the nursing interventions that should be implemented when caring for the monitored woman and her family during labor.

41. A woman is in labor. An external monitor is being used to assess the status of her fetus and the pattern of her uterine contractions. Specify the data that the nurse should document on:
A. Client record

B. Monitor strip

Critical Thinking Exercises

1. Darlene, a primigravida in active labor, has just been admitted to the labor unit. She becomes very anxious when external electronic monitoring equipment is set up. She tells the nurse that her father had a heart attack 2 months ago. "He was so sick they had to put him on a monitor, too. Does this mean that my baby has a heart problem just like my father?" Describe the nurse's expected response.

2. Terry is a primigravida at 43 weeks gestation. Her labor is being stimulated with oxytocin administered intravenously. Her contractions have been increasing in intensity with a frequency of every 2 to 2½ minutes and a duration of 80 to 85 seconds. She is currently in a supine position with a 30-degree elevation of her head. On observation of the monitor tracing, you note that during the last two contractions the FHR decreased after the contraction peaked and did not return to baseline until about 10 seconds into the rest period. A slight decrease in variability and baseline rate was observed.

   A. Identify the pattern described and the possible factors responsible for it.

   B. Describe the actions you would take. State the rationale for each action.

3. Analyze each of the following monitor tracings and document your findings. Describe each FHR pattern depicted and the criteria used to determine if the pattern is reassuring or nonreassuring. Indicate the possible causes, significance, and nursing actions required for each nonreassuring FHR pattern identified.

   A.
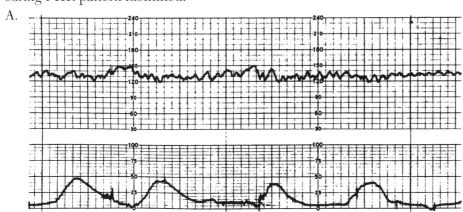

B.

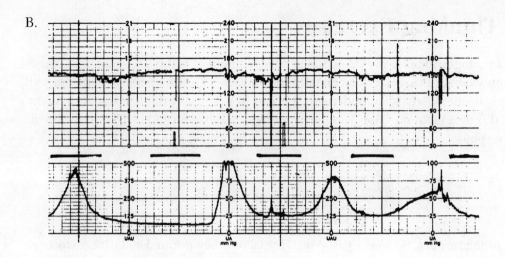

C.

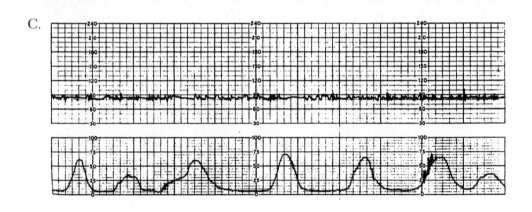

D.

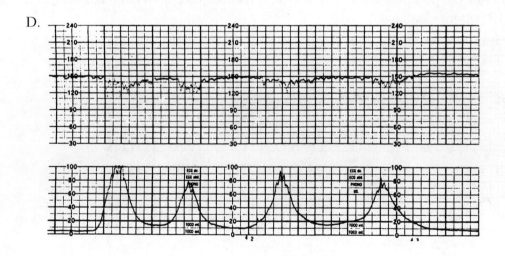

E.

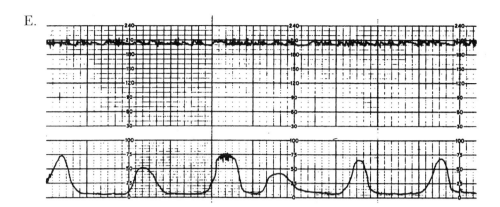

F.

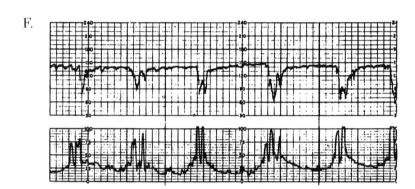

CHAPTER 15

Nursing Care During Labor and Birth

Chapter Review Activities

Evaluate each of the following assessment findings, which are used to distinguish true labor from false labor. Designate whether the assessment finding is associated with true labor (TL) or with false labor (FL).

_____ 1. Contractions regular and progressive

_____ 2. Cervix soft and posterior

_____ 3. Contractions cease with ambulation

_____ 4. Cervix soft, 25%, 2 cm, mid position

_____ 5. Lightening occurs in multiparous woman

_____ 6. Discomfort present in abdomen above umbilicus

_____ 7. Contraction intensity increases with activity and ambulation

_____ 8. Presenting part is above ischial spines

_____ 9. Bloody show

_____ 10. Discomfort radiates from lower back to lower abdomen

_____ 11. Contractions continue even after a shower or backrub

Fill in the Blanks

Insert the term that corresponds to stages of labor for each of the following descriptions.

12. The first stage of labor begins with the onset of _____ and ends with full _____ and _____. A blood-tinged mucous discharge (bloody show) usually indicates the passage of the _____.

13. During the latent phase of the first stage of labor the cervix dilates from _____ to _____ in approximately _____ to _____ hours. Cervical dilatation progresses from _____ to _____ in about _____ to _____ hours during the active phase of the first stage of labor. The duration of the transition phase is approximately _____ minutes and the cervix dilates from _____ to _____.

14. The second stage of labor is the stage when the _____. It begins with full and complete _____. It ends with the _____. This stage is comprised of three phases, namely _____, _____, and _____. The average duration of the second stage of labor for the first pregnancy is _____ and for subsequent pregnancies is _____. A second stage that is longer than _____ in a first pregnancy and longer than _____ in subsequent pregnancies may be considered prolonged in a woman without regional anesthesia and should be reported to the primary health-care provider.

15. The third stage of labor lasts from the time the _____ until the _____. Detachment of the placenta from the wall of the uterus or _____ is indicated by _____, change from a _____ shape to a _____ shape, a sudden _____ from the introitus, apparent _____, and the finding of a _____.

Matching

Match the description in Column I with the appropriate term from Column II.

COLUMN I

_____ 16. Prolonged breath holding while bearing down (closed glottis pushing).

_____ 17. Burning sensation of acute pain as vagina stretches and crowning occurs.

_____ 18. Artificial rupture of membranes (AROM, ARM).

_____ 19. Occurs when widest part of the head (biparietal diameter) distends the vulva just before birth.

_____ 20. Intact amniotic membrane surrounds the newborn's head at birth.

_____ 21. Incision into perineum to enlarge the vaginal outlet.

_____ 22. Test to determine if membranes have ruptured by assessing pH of the fluid.

_____ 23. Technique used to control birth of fetal head and protect perineal musculature.

_____ 24. Expulsion of placenta with fetal side emerging first.

_____ 25. Cord encircles the fetal neck.

_____ 26. Method used to palpate fetus through abdomen.

_____ 27. Occurs when presenting part applies pressure against pelvic floor stretch receptors and results in a woman's perception of an urge to bear down.

_____ 28. Medication that stimulates the uterus to contract.

_____ 29. Expulsion of placenta with maternal surface emerging first.

_____ 30. Protrusion of umbilical cord in advance of the presenting part.

COLUMN II

A. Ritgen's maneuver
B. Episiotomy
C. Oxytocin
D. Ferguson's reflex
E. Shultz mechanism
F. Caul
G. Valsalva's maneuver
H. Ring of fire
I. Crowning
J. Duncan mechanism
K. Amniotomy
L. Nuchal cord
M. Prolapse of umbilical cord
N. Nitrazine test
O. Leopold's maneuvers

Fill in the Blanks

Insert the term that corresponds to the characteristics of the powers of labor for each of the following definitions.

31. _____ The primary powers of labor that act involuntarily to expel the fetus and the placenta from the uterus.

32. _____ "Building up" phase of a contraction.

33. _____ The peak of a contraction.

34. _____ "Letting down" phase of a contraction.

35. _____ How often the contractions occur; the period of time from the beginning of one contraction to the beginning of the next or from the peak of one contraction to the peak of the next.

36. _____ The strength of the contraction at its peak.

37. _____ The period of time that elapses between the onset and end of a contraction.

38. _____ The tension of the uterine muscle during the interval between contractions.

39. _____ Period of rest between contractions.

40. _____ An involuntary urge to push in response to Ferguson's reflex.

41. Assessment of the characteristics and patterns of uterine contractions is an important nursing responsibility.
    A. Label the following illustration that depicts the characteristics of uterine contractions.

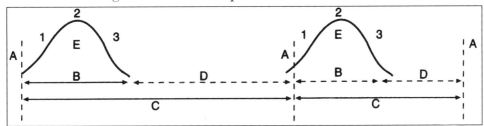

    B. Describe how you would assess each of these characteristics using the palpation method.

42. Laura (3-1-1-0-1) has just been admitted in the latent phase of the first stage of labor. As part of the admission procedure you review her prenatal record, interview her regarding what she has observed regarding her labor, and discuss her current health status.
    A. List the data you would need to obtain from the prenatal record to plan care that is appropriate for Laura.

B. Identify the information required regarding the status of Laura's labor.

C. State the information required regarding Laura's current health status.

True or False

Circle "T" if true or "F" if false for each of the following statements. Correct the false statements.

T F   43. Amniotic fluid will turn Nitrazine test paper greenish-yellow.

T F   44. A partogram is used to diagram the progress of uterine contractions.

T F   45. A laboring woman should be encouraged to void at least every two hours during labor.

T F   46. Ambulation should be encouraged only during the latent phase of the first stage of labor.

T F   47. A hands and knees position is recommended during contractions to facilitate the internal rotation of an occiput posterior position to a more anterior position.

T F   48. The nurse should perform a vaginal examination immediately, using strict sterile technique, if bright red, fresh vaginal bleeding is noted during active labor.

T F   49. Amniotic fluid is alkaline as compared to urine, which is usually acidic.

T F   50. Leopold's maneuvers can assist in the location of the point of maximum intensity (PMI) of the fetal heart beat.

T F   51. Maternal body temperature should be monitored every 1 to 2 hours after the amniotic membranes rupture.

T F   52. Increased sensitivity to touch or hyperesthesia, which develops as labor progresses, results in a woman's rejection of her partner's or the nurse's touch with comfort measures.

T F   53. A woman should begin pushing as soon as the second stage of labor begins.

T F   54. In order for childbirth to progress safely and in a timely fashion, a woman's bearing down efforts must be carefully regulated by the nurse and coach.

T F   55. For pushing to be effective, the woman should maintain a push and hold her breath for at least 10 seconds.

T F   56. The only certain objective sign of the onset of the second stage of labor is the woman's perception of an urge to bear down.

T F   57. During the descent phase of the second stage of labor, pressure of the presenting part on the pelvic floor stimulates release of oxytocin from the pituitary gland thus intensifying uterine contractions.

T F   58. During birth of the head, the woman must continue to fully bear down with uterine contractions to ensure prompt expulsion.

T F   59. If stirrups are used during birth, it is important to place the legs into the stirrups one leg at a time.

T F   60. The time of birth is recorded as the precise time when the newborn takes its first breath.

T F   61. The priority immediately after birth is that the newborn's airway remains patent.

62. Complete the following table by identifying the stressors that a woman and her partner/coach experience during childbirth and the nursing measures that can be supportive and reduce stress.

Woman and partner/coach	Stressors	Support measures
Laboring woman		
Partner/coach		

63. A nurse caring for a laboring woman needs to be alert for signs of potential complications. List these signs.

64. Describe the psychosocial factors that the nurse should observe as the laboring woman progresses through labor.

65. Complete the following table by identifying two advantages for each of the following labor positions.

Labor position	Advantage
Semi-recumbent	
Upright	
Lateral	
Hands and knees	

66. Outline the critical factors to be included in the physical assessment of the maternal-fetal unit during labor.

67. Indicate the laboratory and diagnostic tests that are recommended during labor. State the purpose for each.

68. Complete the following table by identifying two support measures you would use during each phase of the second stage of labor. Validate your response with events and behaviors typical of that phase.

Phase	Events/behaviors	Support measures
Latent		
Descent		
Transition		

69. List the signs that indicate the onset of the second stage of labor.

70. Identify the factors that can influence the duration of the second stage of labor.

71. Describe the maternal positions recommended to enhance the effectiveness of a woman's bearing down efforts during the second stage of labor. State the basis for each position's effectiveness in facilitating the descent and birth of the fetus.

Critical Thinking Exercises

1. Alice, a primigravida, calls the labor unit. She tells the nurse that she thinks she is in labor. "I have had some pains for about two hours. Should my husband bring me to the hospital now?"
   A. Describe how the nurse should approach this situation.

   B. Write several questions the nurse could use to elicit the appropriate information required to determine the course of action required.

   C. Based on the data collected during the telephone interview, the nurse determines that Alice is in very early labor. Since she lives fairly close to the hospital she is instructed to stay home until her labor progresses. Outline the instructions and recommendations for care Alice and her husband should be given.

2. Analyze the assessment findings documented for each of the following women.

Denise	Teresa	Danielle
5 cm	9 cm	2 cm
moderate	very strong	mild
q 4 min	q 2 - 3 min	q 6 - 8 min
40 - 55 sec	65 - 75 sec	30 - 35 sec
0	+2	−1

A. Identify the phase of labor being experienced by each woman.

B. Describe the behavior and appearance you would expect to be exhibited by each woman.

C. Specify the physical care and emotional support measures you would implement if you were caring for each of these women.

3. Describe the procedure that should be followed before auscultating the fetal heart rate or applying an ultrasound transducer to the abdomen of a laboring woman. Explain the rationale for using this procedure.

4. Tonya, a woman in active labor, begins to cry during a vaginal examination to assess her status. "Why not watch the monitor to see how I am progressing instead of doing these vaginal exams? They really hurt and they are embarrassing!"
A. Describe the response the nurse should make to Tonya's concern.

B. Discuss the measures the nurse could use to meet Tonya's safety and comfort needs during a vaginal examination.

5. Tasha is 6 cm dilated. Her coach comes to tell you that her "water just broke with a gush!" Identify each action you would take in this situation, in order of priority. State the rationale for the actions you have identified.

6. Sara, a 17-year-old primigravida, is admitted in the latent phase of labor. Her boyfriend Dan is with her as her only support. They appear committed to each other. During the admission interview, Sara tells you that they did not go to any classes because she was embarrassed about not being married. Both Sara and Dan appear very nervous, and the assessment indicates they know little about what is happening, what to expect, and how to work together with the process of labor. Identify the nursing diagnosis reflected in this data. State one expected outcome and list nursing measures appropriate for the diagnosis you identified.

Nursing diagnosis	**Expected outcome**	**Nursing measures**

7. Identifying a laboring couple's cultural and religious beliefs and practices regarding childbirth is a critical factor in providing culturally sensitive care that enhances the couple's sense of control and eventual satisfaction with their childbirth experience.
   A. List the questions you would ask when assessing a couple's cultural and religious preferences for childbirth.

   B. Discuss the problems that can occur if the nurse does not consider the couple's cultural and religious preferences when planning and implementing care.

8. Cori (4 - 3 - 0 - 0 - 3) is in latent labor. She and her husband are being oriented to the birthing room. Their last birth occurred in a delivery room 10 years ago. Both she and her husband are amazed by the birthing room and the birthing bed that will allow her to give birth in an upright position. They are also informed that changes in bearing down efforts now allow a woman to follow her own body feelings and even to vocalize with pushing. Both Cori and her husband state that with every other birth they put her legs in stirrups, she held her breath for as long as she could, and pushed quietly. "Everything turned out okay so why should we change?" Describe the response the primary nurse caring for this couple should make to their concerns.

9. A nurse living in a rural area is called to her neighbor's home to assist his wife who is in labor. "Everything is happening so fast. She says she is ready to deliver!!"
   A. Identify the measures the nurse can use to reassure and comfort the woman.

   B. Crowning begins shortly after the nurse arrives. State what the nurse should do.

   C. Describe the action the nurse should take after the birth of the head.

   D. List the measures the nurse should use to prevent excessive neonatal heat loss after birth.

   E. Identify the infection control measures that should be implemented during a home birth.

   F. Specify the measures the nurse should use to prevent excessive maternal blood loss or hemorrhage until the ambulance arrives.

G. Outline the information the nurse should document regarding the childbirth.

10. Beth is in the descent phase of the second stage of labor. She is actively pushing and bearing down to facilitate birth. Indicate the criteria a nurse would use to evaluate the correctness of Beth's technique.

11. Molly is entering the second stage of labor. She states that she is experiencing some perineal pressure but refuses to start pushing because as she states, "I am just not ready to push yet."
    A. Discuss the factors that might be inhibiting Molly's desire to bear down and give birth to her baby.

    B. Describe what the nurse could do to help Molly reach the point of readiness to give birth.

12. Imagine that you are participating in a panel discussion on childbirth practices. Your topic is "Episiotomies—are they needed to ensure the safety and well being of the laboring woman and her fetus?" Outline the information you would include in your presentation.

13. Imagine that you are a staff nurse on a childbirth unit. Your hospital is instituting a change in policy that would allow the participation of children in the labor and birth process of their mother. You are asked to be a part of the committee that will formulate the guidelines regarding sibling participation during childbirth. Discuss the suggestions you would make to help ensure a positive outcome for parents, children, and health-care providers.

14. Annie is a primipara in the fourth stage of labor following a long and difficult labor and birth process. She seems disinterested in her baby. Annie looks him over quickly and then asks if you would take him back to the nursery.

    A. Identify the factors that could be accounting for Annie's behavior.

    B. Discuss the nursing measures you would use to encourage future maternal-newborn interactions and facilitate the attachment process.

15. Dawn and Jim's baby was stillborn at 37 weeks gestation. Outline the approach that the nurse caring for this couple should take to help them through the grieving process and form memories of their baby.

CHAPTER 16

Physiologic Changes

Chapter Review Activities

True or False

Circle "T" if true or "F" if false for each of the following statements. Correct the false statements.

T F 1. Within 12 hours of birth the fundus of the uterus may be 1 cm above the umbilicus.

T F 2. The uterus is slightly smaller after every pregnancy.

T F 3. Regeneration of the endometrium, including the placental site, is completed approximately 4 weeks after birth.

T F 4. The weight of a peri pad with lochial flow is 15 grams. This represents a 150 ml blood loss.

T F 5. The external os of the cervix has a jagged, slitlike appearance in multiparous women.

T F 6. Until estrogen levels rise, the postpartum woman is likely to experience discomfort during intercourse (dyspareunia) associated with inadequate secretion of lubricating mucus.

T F 7. The appearance of colostrum is yellowish and thick compared with milk, which appears bluish-white and thin.

T F 8. For most nonlactating women, ovulation resumes by 2 months after birth.

T F 9. During the first 24 hours after birth an elevated temperature of 100.4° F most likely indicates the onset of infection.

T F 10. It is to be expected that the hematocrit level will decrease by the third day postpartum.

T F 11. In the postpartum period a leukocytosis of 20,000/mm^3 strongly indicates uterine or bladder infection.

T F 12. Involution and the process of autolysis often produce a mild proteinuria of +1 for 1 to 2 days after birth.

T F 13. An elevated follicle-stimulating hormone (FSH) in the postpartum period is responsible for the suppression of ovulation in lactating women.

T F 14. The presence of hematuria and edema of the urinary meatus in the early postpartum period following vaginal birth are expected findings.

T F 15. Lochia normally has a fleshy odor similar to menstrual flow.

T F 16. Women with diabetes usually require more insulin for several weeks after they give birth.

17. When caring for a woman following vaginal birth, it is of critical importance for the nurse to assess the woman's bladder for distention.
    A. State why bladder distention is more likely to occur during the immediate postpartum period.

    B. Discuss the problems that can occur if the bladder is allowed to become distended.

18. Identify the factors that can interfere with bowel elimination in the postpartum period.

19. Describe why hypovolemic shock is less likely to occur in the postpartum woman experiencing a normal or average blood loss.

20. Indicate the factors that place a postpartum woman at increased risk for the development of thromboembolism.

21. Contrast the characteristics of lochial bleeding with nonlochial bleeding.

Crossword Puzzle

Postpartum Period

Complete the puzzle after reading Chapters 16, 17, and 18.

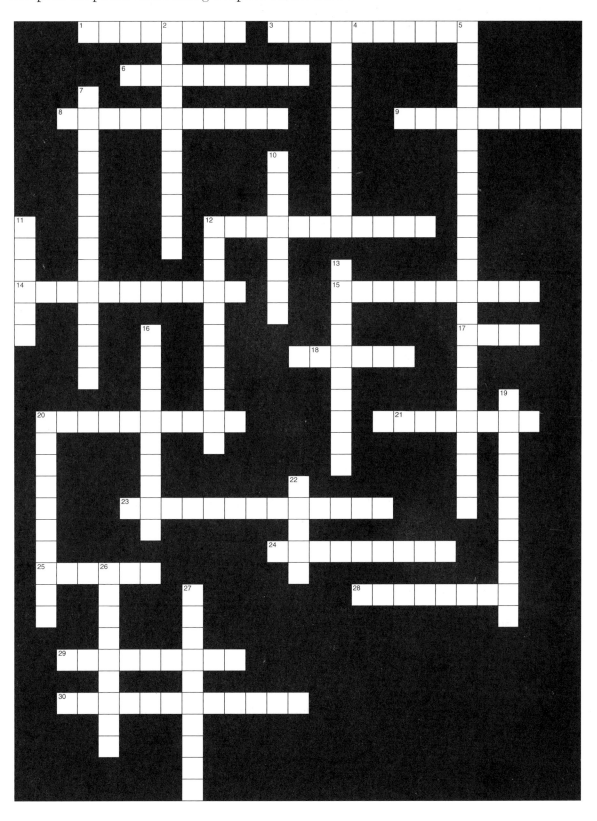

Across

1. Hormone that stimulates the uterus to contract.

3. Period of postpartum maternal adjustment, characterized by vacillation between a need for nurturing and a desire to take charge. (2 words)

6. Process whereby an infant's behaviors and characteristics elicit a corresponding set of maternal behaviors and characteristics.

8. Profuse sweating that occurs after birth, especially at night, to rid the body of fluid retained during pregnancy.

9. The interdependent phase of maternal adjustment in which the resumption of the couple relationship is the major focus. (2 words)

12. The term used to describe the capacity of the newborn to "dance in tune" to the parent's voice.

14. Ability of the infant to turn away from or shut out stimuli.

15. Surgical incision of the perineum to facilitate birth.

17. Term used to describe the yellowish-white lochia that begins about 10 days after birth and continues for 2 to 6 weeks.

18. Term used to describe the pink to brownish colored lochia that begins about 3 to 4 days after birth.

20. Uncomfortable uterine cramping that occurs during the early postpartum period.

21. The identification of the new baby as a member of the family is called the _____ process.

23. Failure of the uterus to fully heal and return to a nonpregnant state. The most common causes are retained placental fragments and infection.

24. The lactogenic hormone produced in large quantities by the pituitary gland of lactating women.

25. Positioning of the infant in a face-to-face, eye-contact position with parent or caregiver.

28. Period of postpartum maternal adjustment characterized by maternal dependency and the need to be nurtured. (2 words)

29. Yellowish fluid produced in the breasts before lactation.

30. Responses that are similar in form to a stimulus behavior, e.g., imitating facial expressions such as smiling.

Down

2. Feeling of dizziness or faintness immediately on standing may be attributed to _____ hypotension.

4. Term used to describe the return of the uterus to a nonpregnant state.

5. Separation of the abdominal wall muscles. (2 words)

7. Term used to describe a person's own pattern of activity.

10. Increased production of urine that occurs in the postpartum period to rid the body of fluid retained during pregnancy.

11. Characteristic uterine discharge after birth.

12. Term used to describe distended, firm, tender, and warm breasts during the postpartum period.

13. An anal varicosity.

16. Term used interchangeably with postpartum to describe the period of recovery following childbirth.

19. The father's absorption, preoccupation, and interest in his infant.

20. Term that describes the feeling of affection and loyalty that binds one person to another, as a parent with a newborn.

22. The bloody lochial flow that occurs for the first few days following birth.

26. A self-destruction process that reduces the size of the uterus after birth by shrinking excess hypertrophied uterine tissue.

27. Postpartum _____ is a more severe form of "baby blues" that is considered to be a type of mental illness that can occur within days of birth or appear gradually up to a year later.

Critical Thinking Exercises

1. Describe how you would respond to each of the following typical questions or concerns of postpartum women.
   A. Mary is a primipara who is breastfeeding. "Why am I experiencing so many painful cramps? I thought this happens only in women who have had babies before."

B. Susan is being discharged after giving birth 20 hours ago. "For how many days should I be able to palpate my uterus to make sure it is firm?"

C. June is a primipara. "My friend, who had a baby last year, said she had a flow for 6 weeks. Isn't that a long time to bleed after having a baby?"

D. Jean is at 24 hours postpartum. "I cannot believe it—I look as if I am still pregnant! How can this be?"

E. Marion is one day postpartum. "I perspired so much last night and I have such large amounts of urine when I go to the bathroom. I hope everything is okay and I can still go home!"

F. Joan is a primipara who is breastfeeding her baby. "My friend told me that I cannot get pregnant as long as I continue to breastfeed. This is great because I do not like to use birth control."

G. Alice, a concerned multiparous woman, states, "My doctor is not going to give me a drug to dry up my breasts like I had with my first baby. How will my breasts ever get back to normal now!"

H. Andrea, a primipara, is one day postpartum. While breastfeeding her baby she confides to the nurse that she does not know how long she will continue to breastfeed. "My husband and I have always had a satisfying sex life but my friend told me that as long as I breastfeed, intercourse is painful."

CHAPTER 17

Assessment and Care During the Fourth Trimester

Chapter Review Activities

Fill in the Blanks

Insert the term that corresponds to the postpartum period for each of the following definitions.

1. _____ The first one to two hours after birth.

2. _____ Nursing care management approach where one nurse cares for both the mother and her infant. It is also called _____ care or _____ care.

3. _____ Classification of medications that stimulates contraction of the uterine smooth muscle.

4. _____ Failure of the uterine muscle to contract firmly. It is the most frequent cause of _____ following childbirth.

5. _____ Treatment that involves sitting in warm water for approximately 20 min to soothe and cleanse the perineal site and to increase blood flow thereby enhancing healing.

6. _____ Menstrual-like cramps experienced by many women when the uterus contracts after childbirth.

7. _____ Tired feeling involving both physiologic components associated with long labors, cesarean birth, anemia, and breastfeeding and psychologic components related to depression and anxiety. This feeling may inhibit the woman's recovery and performance as a mother.

8. _____ Dilatation of the blood vessels supplying the intestines as a result of the rapid decrease in intraabdominal pressure after birth. It causes blood to pool in the viscera and thereby contributes to the development of _____ when the woman who has recently given birth stands up.

9. _____ Complaint of pain in calf muscles when dorsiflexion of the foot is forced. The presence of pain is associated with the presence of a thrombophlebitis.

10. _____ Exercises that can assist women to regain muscle tone that is often lost when pelvic tissues are stretched and torn during pregnancy and birth.

11. _____ Swelling of breast tissue caused by increased blood and lymph supply to the breasts preceding lactation.

12. _____ Vaccine that can be given to postpartum women whose antibody titer is less than 1:8 or whose EIA value is less than 0.79. It is used to prevent nonimmune women from contracting this TORCH infection during a subsequent pregnancy.

13. _____ Also known as RhoGAM, it is given within 72 hr of birth to Rh-negative, antibody (Coombs)-negative women who have Rh-positive newborns. If the fetal screening test is positive in Rh-negative women who give birth to Rh-positive newborns, the _____ test is performed to more accurately determine the amount of fetal blood present in the maternal circulation so that the correct dosage of RhoGAM can be given.

14. State why a woman should breastfeed her newborn during the fourth stage of labor.

15. List measures that can be used to help a postpartum woman to void spontaneously.

16. Identify the measures you would teach a postpartum woman in an effort to prevent the development of thrombophlebitis.

17. State the criteria the nurse should use to determine the progress of a woman's recovery from each of the following types of anesthesia:
    General anesthesia

    Epidural or spinal anesthesia

18. Identify the measures you would teach a mother, who is bottle feeding her infant, to suppress lactation naturally and to relieve discomfort during breast engorgement.

19. State the two most important interventions that can be used to prevent excessive postpartum bleeding in the early postpartum period. Indicate the rationale for the effectiveness of each intervention you identified.

True or False

Circle "T" if true or "F" if false for each of the following statements. Correct the false statements.

T   F   20. The effectiveness of the rubella vaccine may be reduced if a postpartum woman receives both Rh immunoglobulin and a rubella vaccine.

T   F   21. Before sitting in a sitz bath, the woman should relax her gluteal muscles to reduce discomfort when entering the bath, then tighten them after she sits in the bath.

T   F   22. Tucks are used to soothe sore hemorrhoids and perineum.

T   F   23. Medications such as estrogen and Parlodel are no longer used to suppress lactation for the woman who is bottle feeding her infant.

T   F   24. The most dangerous potential complication of the fourth stage of labor is infection.

T   F   25. Ice packs are most effective in minimizing perineal edema during the first 36 hours following birth.

T   F   26. The best time to administer pain medication to a woman who is breastfeeding her infant would be immediately before or after a feeding session.

T   F   27. Rubella vaccine should not be given to a woman who is breastfeeding her infant.

T   F   28. A woman should be expected to void at least 250 ml of urine spontaneously within 2 hr following vaginal birth.

29. Tamara has a midline episiotomy that the nurse must assess.

   A. Describe the position Tamara should assume to facilitate the examination of her episiotomy.

   B. Identify the characteristics that should be assessed to determine progress of healing and adequacy of perineal self-care measures.

30. List the information that the labor/recovery nurse should report to the postpartum nurse when a mother who just gave birth and her baby are transferred to the postpartum unit.

31. Identify the signs of potential complications that may occur during the postpartum period.

Critical Thinking Exercises

1. Tara is breastfeeding her infant 12 hr after delivery. She requests medication for pain. Describe the approach that you would take when fulfilling Tara's request.

2. The nurse notes an excessive rubra flow and early signs of hypovolemic shock in a woman 4 hours after birth.

   A. State the criteria that the nurse should have used to determine that the flow is rubra and excessive, and that the early signs of hypovolemic shock are being exhibited.

   B. Identify the nurse's priority action in response to these assessment findings.

   C. Describe the nurse's legal responsibility in this clinical situation.

   D. Identify additional interventions that a nurse may need to implement to ensure this woman's safety and to prevent the development of further complications.

3. Carrie is a postpartum woman awaiting discharge. Because her rubella titer indicates that she is not immune, a rubella vaccination has been ordered before discharge. State what you would tell Carrie with regard to this vaccination.

4. The physician has written the following order for a postpartum woman: "Administer RhoGAM (Rh immunoglobulin) if indicated." Describe the actions the nurse should take in fulfilling this order.

5. Susan, a postpartum woman, confides to the nurse, "My partner and I have always had a very satisfying sex life even when I was pregnant. My sister told me that this will definitely change now that I have had a baby." Describe what the nurse should tell Susan regarding sexual changes and activity after birth.

6. Identify the priority nursing diagnosis as well as one expected outcome and appropriate nursing management for each of the following situations.
   A. Tina is 2 days postpartum. During a home visit the nurse notes that Tina's episiotomy is edematous, slightly reddened, with approximated wound edges, and no drainage. A distinct odor is noted and there is a buildup of secretions and the Hurricaine gel Tina uses for discomfort. During the interview Tina reveals that she is afraid to wash the area, "I rinse with a little water in my peri bottle in the morning and again at night. I also apply plenty of my gel."

   Nursing diagnosis **Expected outcome** **Nursing management**

B. Erin, who gave birth 3 days ago, has not had a bowel movement since a day or two before labor. She tells the visiting nurse during the interview that she has been avoiding "fiber" foods for fear that the baby will get diarrhea. Her activity level is low. "My family is taking good care of me. I do not have to lift a finger! Besides I would prefer to wait until my episiotomy is less sore before trying to have a bowel movement."

Nursing diagnosis   **Expected outcome**   **Nursing management**

C. Mary gave birth 24 hours ago. She complains of perineal discomfort. "My hemorrhoids and stitches are killing me, but I do not want to take any medication because it will get into my breast milk and hurt my baby."

Nursing diagnosis   **Expected outcome**   **Nursing management**

7. Dawn gave birth 8 hours ago. On palpation, her fundus was two fingerbreadths above the umbilicus and deviated to the right of midline. It was also assessed to be less firm than previously noted.
    A. State the most likely basis for these findings.

    B. Describe the action that the nurse should take based on these assessment findings.

8. Jill gave birth 3 hours ago. During labor, epidural anesthesia was used for pain relief. Jill's primary health-care provider has written the following order, "Out of bed and ambulating when able." Discuss the approach the nurse should take in safely fulfilling this order.

9. Andrea gave birth $1\frac{1}{2}$ hours ago. She tells the nurse that she is ravenous. You check the chart, noting that Andrea's primary health-care provider has ordered "diet as tolerated." State the criteria that should be met before fulfilling this order.

10. Dawn, a primiparous woman at 20 hours postpartum, is preparing for discharge within the next 4 hours. She is breastfeeding her new daughter.
   A. Describe the nurse's legal responsibility in terms of early discharge.

   B. List the criteria for discharge that Dawn and her newborn must meet before discharge from the hospital to home.
   Maternal criteria

   Newborn criteria

   General criteria

   C. Outline the essential content that must be taught before discharge. A home visit by a nurse is planned for Dawn's third postpartum day.

11. Cultural beliefs and practices must be considered when planning and implementing care in the postpartum period.

A. Discuss the importance of using a culturally sensitive approach when providing care to postpartum women and their families.

B. Kim, a Korean-American woman, has just given birth. Assessment reveals that she and her family are guided by beliefs and practices based on a balance of heat and cold. Describe how the nurse would adjust typical postpartum care in order to respect and accommodate Kim's cultural beliefs and practices.

C. A Muslim woman has been admitted to the postpartum unit following the birth of her second son. Describe the approach you would use in managing this woman's care in a culturally sensitive manner.

CHAPTER 18

Adaptation to Parenthood

Chapter Review Activities

1. Complete the following table by identifying the focus, characteristics (typical behaviors and concerns), and care requirements for postpartum women in each of the following phases of maternal adjustment.

Phase	Focus	Characteristics	Care Requirements
Dependent (taking-in)			
Dependent-Independent (taking-hold)			
Interdependent (letting-go)			
Postpartum Blues			

2. Complete the following table by identifying the focus and characteristics (typical behaviors and concerns), and care requirements for fathers in each of the following stages of paternal adjustment to the role of father.

Stage	Focus	Characteristics	Care Requirements
Stage ONE: Expectations			
Stage TWO: Reality			
Stage THREE: Transition to Mastery			

3. Attachment of the newborn to parents and family is critical for optimum growth and development.

   A. Define the process of attachment and bonding.

   B. List conditions that must be present for the parent-newborn attachment process to begin favorably.

   C. Describe the acquaintance process.

4. Identify the six parental tasks and responsibilities that are part of parental adjustment to a new baby.

5. Discuss how each of the following forms of parent-infant contact can facilitate attachment and promote the family as a focus of care.
   Early contact

   Extended contact

6. The parenting process is composed of two essential components. Describe each component and its importance for the optimum growth and development of children. Identify nursing strategies that can be effective in helping parents develop competency and self-confidence with regard to each component.
   Skill/knowledge component   **Valuing/comfort component**

7. During the fourth trimester parents reorganize and modify their roles and relationships as they take on the role of parent to a new baby. State the focus for each period of the fourth trimester:
   Early period (first 3 to 4 weeks)

   Consolidation period

Fill in the Blanks

Insert the appropriate term for each of the following descriptions.

8. The _____ process is the identification of the new baby. The child is first identified in terms of _____ to other family members, then in terms of _____, and finally in terms of _____.

9. _____ is exhibited when newborns move in time with the structure of adult speech by _____, _____, and _____ seemingly _____ to a parent's voice.

10. One of the newborn's tasks is to establish a personal rhythm or _____. Parents can help in this process by giving consistent _____ and using their infant's _____ state to develop _____ behavior and thereby increase _____ and opportunities for _____.

11. _____ is a type of body movement or behavior that provides the observer with cues. The observer or receiver interprets those cues and responds to them. _____ refers to the "fit" between the infant's cues and the parents' response.

12. To modulate _____, both parent and infant must be able to interact. Therefore the infant must be in the _____ state long enough for interactions to take place.

13. The infant and both parents have a _____ of behaviors they can use to facilitate interactions. For the infant these behaviors include _____, _____, and _____. For the parents these behaviors include various types of interactive behaviors such as constantly _____ at the infant and noting the infant's _____. Adults also _____ their speech to help the infant _____. _____ such as slow and exaggerated looks of _____, _____, and _____ are often used by parents to _____ to the infant.

14. Contingent responses or _____ are those that occur within a specific time and are similar in form to a stimulus behavior. The adult has the feeling of having an influence on the interaction. Infant behaviors such as _____, _____, and sustained _____, usually in the _____ position, are viewed as contingent responses.

15. Complete the following table by identifying three infant and parent facilitating behaviors and three infant and parent inhibiting behaviors that can affect the process of attachment.

Infant/Parents	Facilitating Behaviors	Inhibiting Behaviors
Infant		
Parents		

16. Describe how each of the following factors influences the manner in which parents respond to the birth of their child. State two nursing implications/actions related to each factor.

Adolescent parents

Parental age more than 35

Social support

Culture

Socioeconomic conditions

Personal aspirations

Visual impairment

Hearing impairment

Critical Thinking Exercises

1. Jane and Andrew are parents of a newborn girl. Describe what you would teach them regarding the communication process as it relates to their newborn.

   A. Techniques they can use to communicate effectively with their newborn.

   B. The manner in which the baby is able to communicate with them.

2. Allison had a difficult labor that resulted in an emergency cesarean birth under general anesthesia. She did not see her baby until 12 hours after the birth. Allison tells the nurse who brings the baby to her room, "I am so disappointed. I had planned to breastfeed my baby and hold her close, skin-to-skin, right after her birth just like all the books say. I know that this is so important for our relationship." Describe how the nurse should respond to Allison's concern.

3. Angela is the mother of a 1-day-old boy and a 3-year-old girl. As you prepare Angela for discharge, she states, "My little girl just saw her brother. She says she loves him and cannot wait for him to come home. I am so glad that I do not have to worry about any of that sibling rivalry business!" Indicate how you would respond to Angela's comments.

4. Sara and Ben have just experienced the birth of their first baby. They are very happy with their baby boy, but appear unsure of themselves and are obviously anxious about how to tell what their baby needs. Describe what the nurse caring for this family can do to facilitate the attachment process.

5. Mary and Jim are the parents of three sons. They wanted to have a girl this time, but after a long and difficult birth they had another son who weighed 10 pounds. His appearance reflects the difficult birth process: occipital molding, caput succedaneum, and forceps marks on each cheek. Mary and Jim express their disappointment not only in the appearance of their son but also in the fact that they had another boy. "This was supposed to be our last child—now we just do not know what we will do." Discuss how you would facilitate Mary and Jim's attachment to their son and reconcile their fantasy ("dream") child with the reality of their actual child.

6. Dawn and Matthew have just given birth to their first baby. This is the first grandchild for both sets of grandparents. The grandmothers approach the nurse to ask how they can help the new family. "We want to help Dawn and Matthew but at the same time not interfere with what they want to do." Discuss the role of the nurse in helping these grandparents to recognize their importance to the new family and to develop a mutually satisfying relationship with Dawn, Matthew, and the new baby.

7. Jane is two days postpartum. When the nurse makes a home visit, Jane is crying and states, "I have such a let-down feeling. I cannot understand why I feel this way when I should be so happy about the healthy outcome for myself and my baby." Jane's husband confirms her behavior and expresses confusion as well, stating, "I wish I knew what to do to help her." Identify the priority nursing diagnosis and one expected outcome for this situation. Describe the recommended nursing management for the nursing diagnosis you have identified.

Nursing Diagnosis	**Expected Outcome**	**NursingManagement**

CHAPTER 19

Immediate Care of the Newborn

Chapter Review Activities

Neonatal nurses are responsible for the assessment of the physiologic integrity of newborns. As part of this responsibility the nurse must be aware of the significance of data collected. Label each of the following assessment findings, if present in a group of three full-term newborns who were born 12 hours ago, as "**N**" (reflective of normal adaptation or acceptable variation to extrauterine life) or "**P**" (reflective of potential problems with adaptation to extrauterine life).

Assessment Finding	Evaluation
1. Crackles/rales on auscultation of the lungs	_____
2. Respirations: 36, irregular, shallow	_____
3. Episodic apnea lasting 5 to 10 seconds	_____
4. Nasal flaring and sternal retractions	_____
5. Slight bluish discoloration of feet and hands	_____
6. Blood pressure 76/43	_____
7. Apical rate: 126 with murmurs	_____
8. Temperature 37.1° C axillary	_____
9. Head 34 cm and chest 36 cm	_____
10. Boggy, edematous swelling over occiput	_____
11. Overlapping of parietal bones	_____
12. White pimplelike spots on nose and chin	_____
13. Jaundice on face and chest	_____
14. Regurgitation of small amount of milk after feeding	_____
15. Liver palpated 1 cm below right costal margin	_____
16. Absence of bowel elimination since birth	_____
17. Spine straight with dimple at base	_____
18. Adhesion of prepuce—unable to fully retract	_____
19. Edema of scrotum and labia	_____
20. Toes hyperextend/flare when sole is stroked upward	_____
21. Hematocrit 36% and hemoglobin 12 gm/dl	_____
22. White blood cell count (WBC) 23,000/mm^3	_____
23. Blood glucose 45 mg/dl	_____

24. The most critical adjustment that a newborn must make at birth is the establishment of respirations.

    A. List the factors that are responsible for the initiation of breathing after birth.

    B. List the four conditions essential for maintenance of an adequate oxygen supply in the newborn.

    C. Describe the expected respiratory pattern in a newborn.

    D. State four signs that would indicate respiratory distress in the newborn.

    E. Identify three methods of relieving airway obstruction.

25. Complete the following table by identifying the purpose and location of each of the following fetal circulatory shunts and describing the mechanisms responsible for their closure.

Shunt	Purpose/Location	Closure Mechanism
Foramen ovale		
Ductus arteriosus		
Ductus venosus		

26. Cold stress presents a danger if experienced by the newborn during the postbirth period.
    A. List the dangers the newborn faces if he or she experiences cold stress.

    B. Identify the characteristic newborn behaviors associated with cold stress.

    C. Identify several measures the nurse can use to stabilize a newborn's temperature.

    D. State three guidelines the nurse should follow when placing a newborn under a radiant heat panel.

27. Complete the following table by defining each of the following heat loss mechanisms and identifying one nursing measure that can be used to prevent heat loss as a result of each mechanism.

Heat Loss Mechanism	Definition of Heat Loss Mechanism	Nursing Measure to Prevent Heat Loss
Convection		
Radiation		
Evaporation		
Conduction		

28. Identify the specific criteria or assessment findings that characterize physiologic jaundice.

Fill in the Blanks: Behavioral Adaptations of the Newborn

Insert the appropriate term for each of the following descriptions.

29. Variations in the state of consciousness of newborn infants are called the _____-states. The sleep states are _____ sleep and _____ sleep. The wake states are _____, _____, _____, and _____. The optimum state of arousal is the _____ state in which the infant can be observed _____, _____, _____, _____, and _____. The infant's reactions to _____ and _____ stimuli and ability to control their _____ while in these states reflect their ability to _____.

30. During the first 6 to 8 hours after birth, newborns experience a transitional period characterized by three phases of instability. Complete the following table by identifying the timing and duration and typical behaviors for each phase.

Phase	Timing/Duration	Typical Behaviors
First Period of Reactivity		
Period of Diminished Response		
Second Period of Reactivity		

31. Identify two nursing measures that can be used to limit the degree of physiologic hyperbilirubinemia. State the basis for the effectiveness of each measure identified.

32. State the nurse's legal responsibility regarding identification of the newborn at birth.

True or False

Circle "T" if true or "F" if false for each of the following statements. Correct the false statements.

T   F   33. The presence of phosphatidylglycerol (Pg) in amniotic fluid is more predictive of fetal lung maturity that is an L/S ratio (lecithin/sphingomyelin) of 2:1.

T   F   34. Crackles, grunting, nasal flaring, and retractions are often noted during the first and second periods of reactivity.

T   F   35. The white blood cell count of the newborn will not increase markedly and may even decline in infection.

T   F   36. Vitamin B_{12} is often given intravenously to newborns immediately after birth to enhance clotting and prevent hemorrhage.

T   F   37. Blood-tinged mucus on the diaper of the female newborn should be documented by the nurse as pseudomenstruation and recognized as an expected assessment finding related to the withdrawal of maternal hormones.

T   F   38. Physiologic jaundice in the full-term newborn appears after the first 24 hours of life and disappears by the end of the first week of life.

T   F   39. Breastfeeding jaundice commonly appears about the third day of life, whereas breast milk jaundice appears after the first week of life.

T   F   40. Kernicterus, the most severe complication of neonatal hyperbilirubinemia, occurs when bilirubin invades the cells of the heart muscle thereby weakening heart function.

T   F   41. Chest movements are counted when determining the respiratory rate of newborns since breathing is primarily thoracic in nature.

T   F   42. A drop of 20 mm Hg in the systolic blood pressure is an expected finding during the first hour after birth.

T   F   43. Meconium stool often has a strong odor as a result of bacteria present in the fetal intestine during intrauterine life.

T   F   44. Breast tissue in full-term male and female newborns may be swollen and secrete a thin milky-type discharge.

T   F   45. CPR for infants recommends cycles of five compressions and one ventilation (a 5:1 ratio) with the fifth compression completed in 3 seconds or less.

T   F   46. A delay of up to two hours of instilling a prophylactic agent into a newborn's eyes is acceptable to facilitate parent-infant attachment and bonding.

T   F   47. If an infant's airway is obstructed by a foreign body, the infant should receive three chest thrusts followed by two back blows.

T   F   48. Placing a dressed newborn under a radiant heat panel facilitates a rapid stabilization of body temperature after birth.

T   F   49. The thermistor probe of a radiant heat panel should be taped to the right upper quadrant of the abdomen just below the intercostal margin (ribs).

T   F   50. For the first 12 hours after birth, a newborn's temperature should be taken rectally until stabilized because it is more accurate.

T   F   51. Penicillin ointment is instilled into the newborn's lower conjunctiva to prevent ophthalmia neonatorum.

Crossword Puzzle: The Newborn

Complete the following puzzle after reading Chapters 19, 20, and 21.

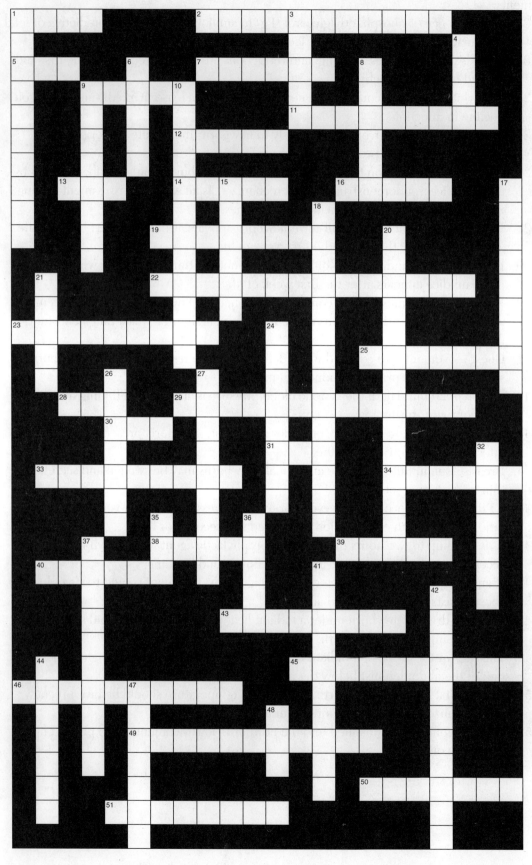

Across

1. Reflex action produced when a finger is placed in the newborn's mouth.

2. Protective mechanism that allows the infant to become accustomed to environmental stimuli.

5. Breakdown of the _____, known as hemolysis, often results in hyperbilirubinemia of the newborn.

7. Space between neonatal skull bones.

9. White facial pimples caused by distended sebaceous glands.

11. Reflex that automatically pushes food out of the mouth when it is placed on the newborn's tongue.

12. Wrinkles/skin folds on the scrotum.

13. Number of veins in the umbilical cord.

14. Intestinal cramps related to a reduction in gastric acidity.

16. Pink or rust stains left on a diaper by uric acid crystals in the urine are often called _____ dust.

19. Yellowish skin discoloration caused by increased levels of indirect or unconjugated bilirubin.

22. Bluish-black pigmented areas usually found on back and buttocks. (two words)

23. Color variation related to vasoconstriction on one side of the body and vasodilation on the other; it occurs when the infant lies on its side and the lower half of the body becomes pink while the upper half is pale.

25. Symmetric _____ folds of the buttocks are one indicator of proper hip placement.

28. Number of arteries in the umbilical cord.

29. White, cheeselike protective substance found on the skin at birth.

30. Designation for newborns who exceed the weight standard for their gestational age.

31. Designation for newborns who fall short of the weight standard for their gestational age.

33. When supine, newborn's arm will extend on the side toward which the head is turned and the opposite arm will flex. (two words)

34. Transient, spontaneous motor activity or quivering noted when in an alert state or during episodes of crying.

38. Reflexive response of fingers when an object is placed in the palm.

39. Shunt between the two atria is the foramen _____.

40. White, cheeselike substance found under the prepuce and between the labia.

43. Specialized adipose tissue used for thermogenesis. (two words)

45. Substance that facilitates expansion and stability of alveoli, thereby enhancing respiration.

46. Flow of heat from body surface to cooler ambient air.

49. Heat loss through vaporization of moisture from the skin.

50. Desquamation present at birth in a postterm neonate.

51. Appearance and disappearance of primitive newborn _____ reflect neurologic integrity and state of neurologic maturation.

Down

1. Transient cross-eyed appearance lasting until the third or fourth month of life.

3. Total number of blood vessels in the umbilical cord.

4. Startle response to a sudden, intense stimulus.

6. Nares will _____ when respiratory distress is present.

8. Transitory cardiac sound produced when blood flows through the incompletely closed fetal shunts such as the foramen ovale.

9. Thick, green-black stool usually passed within 24 hr of birth.

10. Bluish discoloration of the hands and feet.

15. Soft downy hair on face, shoulders, and back.

17. Accumulation of fluid around the testes.

18. Pinkish areas on upper eyelids, nose, upper lip, back of head, and neck known as stork bites or nevi.

20. Collection of blood between skull bone and its periosteum as a result of pressure during birth.

21. Small, white epithelial cyst on the midline of the hard palate known as an Epstein's _____.

24. Hyperextension of toes with an upward stroke on the sole indicates a positive _____ reflex.

26. Overlapping of cranial bones to facilitate passage of the fetal head through the maternal pelvis during the birth process.

27. Red pinpoint marks most often related to pressure applied to the presenting part or area of the body during the birth process.

32. Turn of head and opening of mouth when a hungry newborn is touched on the cheek or corner of the mouth.

35. Designation for newborns who meet the weight standard for their gestational age.

36. Method for assessment of newborn at 1 and 5 minutes after birth is called the _____ score.

37. Phases of the transition to extrauterine life include the first and second periods of _____.

41. Heat loss from body surface to cooler surface with which it is in direct contact.

42. Reflex that stimulates peristalsis during or just after a feeding.

44. Erythema _____ is a sudden, transient newborn rash characterized by erythematous macules, papules, or small vesicles.

47. Lines or wrinkles on the soles of the feet indicative of maturity.

48. A fat or sucking _____ gives each cheek a full appearance and serves to facilitate feeding.

Critical Thinking Exercises

1. Apgar scoring is a method of newborn assessment used immediately after birth, at one and 5 minutes. Indicate the Apgar score for each of the following newborns.

   Baby boy Smith at 1 minute after birth:
   Heart rate: 120 beats per minute
   Respiratory effort: good, crying vigorously
   Muscle tone: active movement
   Reflex irritability: cries with stimulus to soles of feet
   Color: body pink, hands and feet cyanotic
   Score: _____
   Interpretation:

   Baby girl Doe at 5 minutes after birth:
   Heart rate: 102 beats per minute
   Respiratory effort: slow, irregular
   Muscle tone: some flexion of extremities
   Reflex irritability: grimace with stimulus to soles of feet
   Color: pale, as the fifth apgar score finding
   Score: _____
   Interpretation:

2. Significant variations occur in physiologic functioning of the newborn and adult. Complete the following table by identifying these variations and the implications for newborn care.

Physiologic Function	Variations	Implications for Care
Respiratory Patterns		
Cardiovascular Patterns		
Thermoregulation		
Hematopoietic Characteristics		
Renal Function		

3. After a long and difficult labor, baby boy James was born with a caput succedaneum, a single small cephalhematoma on the left parietal bone, and significant molding over the occipital area. Low forceps were used for the birth, resulting in ecchymotic areas on both cheeks. Describe what you would tell the parents of James about these assessment findings.

4. Tonya and Sam, an African-American couple, express concern that their new baby girl has several bruises on her back and buttocks. They ask if their baby was injured during birth or in the nursery. Describe the appropriate response of the nurse to Tonya and Sam's concern.

5. Baby girl Brown has an accumulation of mucus in her nasal passages and mouth, making breathing difficult.
   A. State the nursing diagnosis represented by the assessment findings.

   B. List the steps that the nurse should follow when clearing the baby's airway with a bulb syringe.

   C. If mucous accumulation continues and breathing is compromised, a nasopharyngeal catheter with mechanical suction may be required. List the guidelines a nurse should follow when using this method to clear the newborn's airway.

6. Baby girl June was just born.
   A. Outline the protocol the nurse should follow when assessing June's physical status during the first 2 hours after her birth.

   B. State two priority nursing diagnoses appropriate for June during the first 2 hours after birth.

   C. Identify the priority nursing care measures that the nurse must implement to ensure June's well-being and safety during the first 2 hours after birth.

7. Angie tells the nurse that she is a little worried about breastfeeding her 1-day-old baby boy. "My best friend breastfed her baby and the baby turned yellow and had to stay in the hospital for an extra day after she went home." Describe an appropriate response of the nurse to Angie's concern.

CHAPTER 20

Assessment and Care of the Newborn

Chapter Review Activities

True or False

Circle "T" if true or "F" if false for each of the following statements. Correct the false statements.

T F 1. Tympanic thermometers should not be used until after the first month of life.

T F 2. After a feeding, the infant should be placed on its right side to facilitate gastric emptying into the small intestine.

T F 3. Both breastfed and bottle-fed babies should be fed every 3 to 4 hours during the day and through the night.

T F 4. The recommended site for an intramuscular injection in the newborn is the vastus lateralis muscle.

T F 5. If bleeding is noted after a circumcision, the nurse should apply firm, constant pressure to the site until the physician arrives.

T F 6. To facilitate obtaining a heel stick blood sample, the loose application of a warm wet washcloth around the foot for 5 to 10 minutes is sufficient to dilate the blood vessels in the heel.

T F 7. An alcohol swab should be used to apply pressure to the heel after a blood sample is obtained.

T F 8. Pressure should be applied over an arterial or femoral vein puncture for at least 5 minutes to prevent bleeding from the site.

T F 9. Before applying a U-Bag, the genitalia, perineum, and surrounding skin should be washed, dried, and sprinkled with talcum powder to prevent excoriation.

T F 10. For a single void specimen, 1 to 2 ml of urine are required.

T F 11. Nonnutritive sucking with a pacifier or finger should be discouraged in the newborn because it leads to malformation of the jaw and to dependency.

T F 12. An expected newborn blood glucose level should be between 45 and 90 mg/dl.

T F 13. Hepatitis B vaccine should only be administered to newborns exposed to the hepatitis B virus.

T F 14. The prone position should not be used for the first few months of life since it has been associated with an increase in the risk for sudden infant death syndrome (SIDS).

T F 15. A newborn usually loses approximately 10% of its birth weight during the first few days of life as a result of fluid loss, limited fluid intake, and an increased metabolic rate.

T F 16. Postterm infants are considered to be large for gestational age.

T F 17. A preterm infant could be considered appropriate for gestational age if its rate of growth was normal during fetal life.

T   F   18. A difference of 10 mm Hg or greater in blood pressure between the upper and lower extremities is an acceptable finding in newborns.

T   F   19. The wink reflex can be used to assess anal patency.

T   F   20. Congenital hypothyroidism is diagnosed by testing the newborn for low levels of T_3 and TSH.

Fill in the Blanks

Insert the appropriate term into each blank.

21. _____ can be used to assess for hip dysplasia by listening for a clicking sound when the legs are abducted.

22. _____ is administered to the newborn intramuscularly in a single dose of _____ after birth to prevent hemorrhagic disorders. A _____ gauge, _____-inch needle is used when administering intramuscular injections such as the hepatitis B vaccine and Vitamin K to newborns.

23. During a circumcision the _____ of the glans penis is removed. If properly performed it prevents _____ a rare condition that can impede the flow of urine and predispose males to the development of infection between the _____ and the _____. The risk of _____ and _____ may also be reduced as a result of circumcision. The decision to perform this elective procedure is left up to the _____.

24. _____ is the ability of the infant to respond to and then inhibit responding to discrete stimuli (light, rattle, bell, pinprick) while asleep. It is a protective mechanism that allows the infant to be accustomed to _____. It is a psychologic and physiologic phenomenon whereby the response to a _____ or _____ stimulus is _____.

25. _____ is the quality of alert states and the ability to attend to visual and auditory stimuli when alert.

26. _____ is the measure of general arousal level or arousability of the infant whereas _____ refers to how the infant responds when aroused.

27. _____ refers to quality of movement and muscle tone.

28. _____ refers to signs of stress such as tremors, startles, and skin color related to homeostatic (self-regulator) adjustment of the nervous system.

29. _____ refers to the ability of newborns to comfort themselves or to be comforted by others. In the crying state, most newborns initiate one of several ways to reduce their distress including _____ as well as _____ to _____, _____, or _____ stimuli.

30. _____ refers to the ability of newborns to mold into the contours of the persons holding them.

31. The most widespread use of postnatal testing for genetic disease is the routine screening of newborns for _____ which are a large group of disorders caused by a metabolic defect that results from the absence of or change in a protein, usually an enzyme, and mediated by the action of a certain gene. One example of this type of disorder is _____, which results from a deficiency of the enzyme phenylalanine dehydrogenase. Before testing for this disorder, the nurse must document the initial ingestion of _____ and then perform the test at least _____ after that time. _____ is a disorder that results in the inability to convert galactose to _____. If this disorder goes untreated the infant will exhibit _____, _____, _____, _____, _____, and _____. The same blood sample can be used to test for both disorders as well as _____.

32. The new Ballard scale is used to assess clinical gestational age of the newborn.
   A. List the signs assessed to determine neuromuscular maturity. Indicate the expected finding for a full-term newborn for each sign listed.

   B. List the signs assessed to determine physical maturity. Indicate the expected finding for a full-term newborn for each sign listed.

   C. For an infant with a gestational age of 20 weeks or less the examination should be performed at a postnatal age of less than _____ hours. For an infant with a gestational age of at least 26 weeks the examination can be performed up to _____ hours after birth.

   D. Explain how the designations of AGA, SGA, and LGA are made.

33. Preparing parents for the discharge of their newborn requires informing them about the essential aspects of newborn care. Identify the information you would teach parents regarding each of the following areas:
   Umbilical cord

   Positioning and holding a newborn

   Airway patency

   Temperature

Elimination

Bathing

34. List the safety and medical aseptic principles that should be followed when sponge bathing a newborn.

35. Describe how each of the following factors can influence a newborn's behavior.
Gestational age

Time

Stimuli

Medication

Ethnicity

Sensory behaviors

36. Complete the following table by identifying the stimulus and expected response for each of the reflexes listed.

Newborn Reflex	Stimulus	Expected Response
Rooting		
Grasp (palmar, plantar)		
Extrusion		
Glabellar		
Tonic neck		
Moro		
Stepping/Walking		
Babinski's sign		
Pull-to-sit (traction)		

Continued

Newborn Reflex	Stimulus	Expected Response
Trunk incurvature		
Magnet		

37. Specify the guidelines a nurse should follow when weighing and measuring the newborn to ensure accuracy of the finding and safety of the newborn.

Weight

Head circumference

Chest circumference

Abdominal circumference

Length

38. The Brazelton Neonatal Behavioral Assessment Scale (BNBAS) and Mother's Assessment of the Behavior of her Infant (MABI) are often used to assess newborns.

A. State the purpose of these assessment scales.

B. List the clusters of neonatal behavior assessed using the BNBAS.

39. Describe how the nurse would meet the prescribed standards for a newborn protective environment in terms of each of the following areas:

Environment

Infection control

Safety

Critical Thinking Exercises

1. Baby boy Jones is 20 hours old. The nurse will perform a physical examination of this newborn before he is discharged.
   A. Identify information from the maternal health history and the prenatal and intrapartal records the nurse should gather before the newborn's examination.

   B. List the actions the nurse should take to ensure safety and accuracy during the physical examination. Include the rationale for the actions identified.

   C. Identify the major points that should be assessed as part of this physical examination.

D. Support the premise that Baby boy Jones' parents should be present during this examination.

2. Susan and James are taking their newly circumcised (6 hours after the procedure) baby home. This is their first baby and they express anxiety concerning care of both the circumcision and the umbilical cord.
   A. State one nursing diagnosis related to this situation.

   B. State one expected outcome related to the nursing diagnosis identified.

   C. Specify the instructions that the nurse should give to Susan and James regarding assessment of both sites and the care measures required to facilitate healing.

3. Mary and Jim are concerned that their 2-day-old baby boy, who weighed 8 pounds and 6 ounces at birth, now weighs "only 7 pounds and 14 ounces." Describe how the nurse should respond to Mary and Jim's concern about their baby's weight loss.

4. Andrew and Marion are parents of a newborn, 30 hours old, who has developed hyperbilirubin-emia. They are very concerned about the color of their baby and the need to put the baby under special lights. "Andrew's uncle was yellow just like our baby and later died of liver cancer!"
   A. Describe how the nurse should respond to Andrew and Marion's concern.

B. Identify the expected assessment findings and physiologic effects related to hyperbilirubine-mia.

C. List the precautions and care measures required by the newborn undergoing phototherapy in order to prevent injury to the newborn yet maintain the effectiveness of the treatment. State the rationale for each action identified.

5. Lara and Troy are first time parents of a baby girl. They ask the nurse about their baby's ability to see and hear things around her and to interact with them.
   A. Specify what the nurse should tell Lara and Troy about the sensory capabilities of their healthy full-term daughter.

   B. Name four stimuli that Lara and Troy could provide their baby to facilitate her development.

6. Sheila is a 21-year-old single woman who just gave birth to her first child by cesarean section. It is important for the nurse to assess the process of parent-infant attachment.
   A. Describe five attachment behaviors that the nurse would observe when Sheila and her baby are together.

   B. Identify several factors that can influence the development of attachment and parenting.

CHAPTER 21

Newborn Nutrition and Feeding

Chapter Review Activities

1. Calculate the daily energy (kcal), and fluid requirements for each of the following newborns.

Infant	Calories	Fluid
Jim: 1 month 4 kg		
Sue: 4 months 6 kg		
Sam: 7 months 7.5 kg		

2. Label the following illustration as indicated:

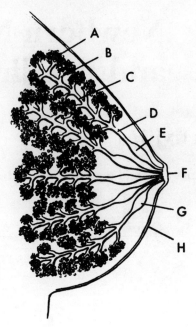

Lactation structures of the female breast

3. Identify the advantages of breastfeeding for each of the following.
Infant

Mother

Families and society

4. Describe four recommended breastfeeding positions.

5. Infants exhibit feeding readiness cues as they recognize and express their hunger.
   A. Identify feeding readiness cues of the infant.

   B. State why the new mother should be guided by these cues when determining the timing of feeding sessions.

6. Indicate the difference between foremilk and hindmilk.

7. Label each of the following illustrations depicting the maternal breastfeeding reflexes.

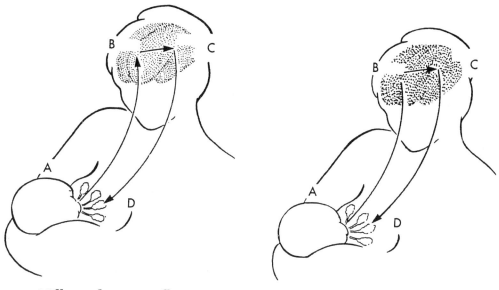

Milk production reflex   **Let-down reflex**

8. There are three stages of lactogenesis. State expected time of occurrence for each stage and describe the events typical of each stage.
   Stage I

Stage II

Stage III

9. State the AWHONN guidelines for breastfeeding support during pregnancy and following birth.

10. Proper latch-on is essential for effective breastfeeding and preservation of nipple/areolar tissue integrity.

   A. Indicate the steps a woman should follow to ensure a proper latch-on.

   B. Describe the signs indicative of a proper latch-on.

True or False

Circle "T" if true or "F" if false for each of the following statements. Correct the false statements.

T   F   11. Approximately 75% of infants in the United States are breastfed.

T   F   12. The most significant increase in breastfeeding is among well-educated, upper income, Caucasian women.

T   F   13. A newborn should lose no more than 10% of its birth weight.

T   F   14. The birth weight of a full-term newborn is usually regained within 10 to 14 days of life.

T   F   15. To prevent fat-related cardiovascular problems later in life, infants should be given low fat or skim milk after the first 6 months of life if they are not being breastfed.

T   F   16. Infants who are entirely breastfed should receive iron supplementation in the form of iron-containing foods such as cereals after the first 6 months of life.

T   F   17. Women who have large breasts will produce more milk than women who have small breasts.

T   F   18. Milk production depends primarily on prolactin secretion and efficient emptying of the breasts.

T F 19. Women from some cultures avoid breastfeeding until the milk comes in since they believe that colostrum is unclean and may harm the baby.

T F 20. Early and frequent feeding facilitates the elimination of bilirubin in feces, thereby reducing the incidence or severity of hyperbilirubinemia and jaundice.

T F 21. Diabetic women should avoid breastfeeding since insulin requirements are increased.

T F 22. Colostrum acts as a laxative to remove meconium from the newborn's intestine.

T F 23. Breastfed babies require vitamin C supplementation.

T F 24. Nicotine can inhibit the letdown reflex.

T F 25. When breastfeeding a newborn, pacifiers should be avoided for the first few weeks until the newborn becomes proficient with breastfeeding.

T F 26. Uterine cramping with or without an increase in lochial flow indicates that oxytocin is being secreted during breastfeeding.

T F 27. Fluoride supplementation should begin at 2 months for breastfed and bottle-fed babies not receiving fluoridated water.

T F 28. A woman with mastitis should stop breastfeeding temporarily as soon as the diagnosis of infection is made.

29. Identify several techniques that can be used to calm a fussy, crying baby in preparation for feeding.

30. Complete the following table by identifying the factors that should be assessed before and during breastfeeding and the factors for ongoing assessment as related to the infant and the breastfeeding mother.

Infant/Mother	Assessment Before and During Breastfeeding	Ongoing Assessment
INFANT		
MOTHER		

Crossword Puzzle: Lactation

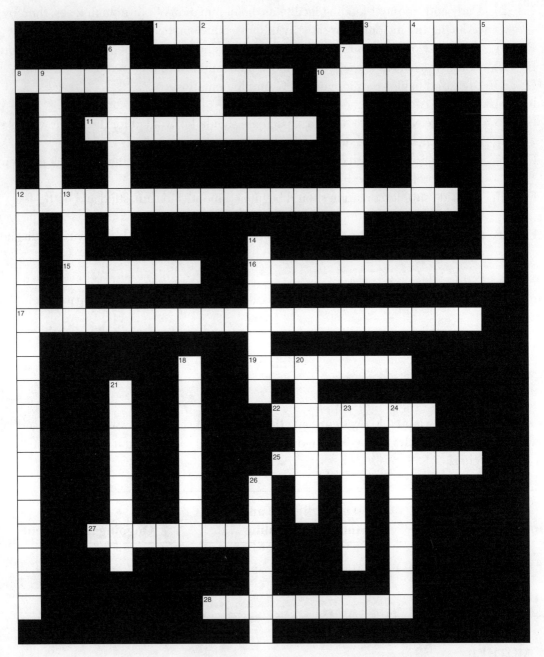

Across

1. Infection of the breast that may be manifested by a swollen, tender breast and sudden onset of flu-like symptoms.

3. Manual application of gentle but deep pressure to the breasts in order to trigger the let-down reflex and facilitate expression of milk.

8. The process of milk production.

10. Exposing the newborn to both breast and bottle nipples can lead to nipple _____, a difficulty in knowing how to latch on to the breast after having taken a bottle.

11. Structures in the breast that are composed of alveoli, milk ductules, and myoepithelial cells. (two words)

12. Professional who specializes in breastfeeding and may be available to assist a new mother with breastfeeding while in the hospital or after discharge. (two words)

15. Once the baby is gaining weight properly, the baby can determine the timing of its own feedings. This is often referred to as _____ feeding.

16. Occurs around the third or fourth day, when an increased volume of milk fills the breasts, which then become tender, swollen, hot and hard, and even shiny and red.

17. Newborn behaviors that indicate hunger and a desire to eat. (three words)

19. Process whereby the infant is gradually introduced to drinking from a cup and eating solid food while breastfeeding is reduced by gradually decreasing the number of feedings.

22. An _____ nipple becomes hard and erect, and protrudes upon stimulation thereby facilitating latch on.

25. Very concentrated, high-protein, antibody-rich substance present in the breasts before the formation of milk.

27. Breast structure that connects several alveoli. (two words)

28. Hormone secreted from the anterior pituitary gland in response to the infant's suck and emptying of the breast.

Down

2. A breast _____ is a plastic device that can be placed over the nipple and areola to keep clothing off the nipple and put pressure around the base of the nipple to promote eversion or protrusion of the nipple.

4. At times infants do not respond to stimulation and withdraw into sleep even after several attempts to awaken them for feeding. This behavior is termed _____.

5. A period lasting about 48 hours when the infant will be fussy and desire to eat more often than usual. Milk production will increase in response to demand. (two words)

6. An infection that is caused by a fungus, the organism that causes thrush in the newborn's mouth. Both of the mother's nipples and the baby's mouth must be treated simultaneously.

7. For the _____ position, the mother holds the baby's back and shoulders in her hand with the baby's body tucked under the arm.

9. Rounded, pigmented section of tissue surrounding the nipple.

12. Milk collection structures that narrow to form the many openings in the nipple. They are compressed with infant sucking and the milk is ejected. (two words)

13. For the _____ position, the baby's head is positioned in the crook of the arm and the mother and baby are "tummy-to-tummy."

14. The _____ reflex, also known as the milk ejection reflex, is triggered by the contraction of myoepithelial cells. Colostrum and later milk are ejected toward the nipple. (two words)

18. An _____ nipple remains flat and soft and does not protrude or evert even with stimulation.

20. Clusters of milk-producing cells.

21. Hormone secreted by the posterior pituitary. It triggers the milk ejection reflex.

23. The _____ reflex is stimulated when a hungry baby's mouth or lips are touched. The baby opens its mouth and begins to suck.

24. A newborn will automatically push solid food out of its mouth when the food is placed on its tongue as a result of the _____ reflex.

26. Positioning of the baby onto the breast when its mouth is open wide and tongue is down. The nipple and some of the areola should be in the baby's mouth. (two words)

Critical Thinking Exercises

1. Evaluate each of the following actions of Janet, a breastfeeding mother. Determine if the action indicates competency (+) or a need for further instruction (−). Indicate what information you would give Janet to correct actions that require further instruction.
   ____ A. Washes her breasts thoroughly with soap and water twice a day.
   ____ B. Massages a small amount of breast milk into her nipple and areola before and after each feeding.
   ____ C. Inserts a thick plastic-lined pad into her bra to absorb leakage.
   ____ D. Positions baby supporting back and shoulders securely and then brings her breast toward the baby, putting the nipple in its mouth.
   ____ E. Alternates breastfeeding positions among football, cradle, modified cradle, and lying down holds.
   ____ F. Limits breastfeeding at the first breast to a maximum of 10 minutes then switches to the second breast.
   ____ G. Supports her breast with four fingers underneath the breast and thumb on the top at the back edge of the areola.
   ____ H. Inserts her finger into the corner of her baby's mouth between the gums before removing the infant from her breast.
   ____ I. Awakens the baby every 2 to 3 hours day and night to feed.
   ____ J. Increases her fluid intake to 3 L/day by drinking water, coffee, juice, milk, cola, wine, and beer.
   ____ K. Increases her caloric intake by 500 calories each day with a gradual weight loss noted.
   ____ L. Plans to use the "pill" for birth control beginning at 3 weeks postpartum.

2. Tonya is bottle feeding her baby. She expresses concern to the nurse at the well-baby clinic about heart disease and cholesterol levels as they relate to her 2-month-old baby. She tells the nurse that her family has a history of cardiac disease and hypertension and she has already changed her diet and wants to do the same for her baby. Tonya asks, "When should I start giving my baby skim milk instead of the prepared formula that I am using which seems to contain quite a bit of fat?" Discuss how the nurse should respond to Tonya's question.

3. Elise and her husband Mark are experiencing their first pregnancy. During one of their prenatal visits, they tell the nurse that they are as yet unsure about the method they want to use for feeding their baby. "Everyone has an opinion. Some say breastfeeding is best, yet others tell us that bottle feeding is more convenient especially since the father can help. What should we do?"
   A. Discuss why is it important for the pregnant couple to make this decision together.

   B. Indicate why is it preferable to make this decision during the prenatal period rather than waiting until the baby is born.

   C. Describe how the nurse could use the decision-making process to assist Elise and Mark to choose the method that is best for them.

4. Mary, as a first time breastfeeding mother, has many questions. Describe how you would respond to the following questions and comments.
   A. "I am so afraid that I will not make enough milk for my baby. My breasts are not as large as some of my friends who breastfeed."

   B. "Everyone keeps talking about this let down that is supposed to happen. What is it and how will I know I have it?"

   C. "How can I possibly know if breastfeeding is going well and my baby is getting enough if I cannot tell how many ounces he gets with each feeding?"

   D. "It is only the first day that I am breastfeeding and my nipples already feel sore. What can I do to relieve this soreness and prevent it from getting worse?"

E. "My friends all told me to watch out for the fourth day and engorgement. What can I do to keep it from happening or at least take care of myself when it does?"

F. "Every time I breastfeed, I get cramps and my flow seems to get heavier. Is there something wrong with me?"

G. "I am so glad I do not have to worry about getting pregnant again as long as I am breastfeeding. I hate using birth control and my friend told me I do not have to as long as I am breastfeeding!"

H. "What should I do when I am ready to stop feeding my baby?"

5. Before discharge with her healthy, full-term baby boy, Jane, a primiparous woman, asks the nurse about when she should start solid foods like cereals, "so that the baby will sleep through the night?" Describe how the nurse should respond to Jane's request for information.

6. Susan is 1 day old and was last fed 5 hours ago. Her mother tells the nurse that Susan is so sleepy that she just does not have the heart to wake her. Discuss the approach the nurse should take with regard to this situation.

7. Alice has decided that for personal and professional reasons, bottle feeding with a commercially prepared formula is the feeding method that is best for her. She tells the nurse that she hopes she made a good decision for her baby. "I hope she will be well nourished and feel that I love her even though I am bottle feeding."
   A. Describe how the nurse should respond to Alice's concern.

   B. State three guidelines for bottle-feeding technique that the nurse should teach Alice to ensure the safety and health of her baby.

CHAPTER 22

Assessment for Risk Factors

Chapter Review Activities

True or False

Circle "T" if true or "F" if false for each of the following statements. Correct the false statements.

T   F   1. In 1996, the lowest infant mortality rate in the United States was recorded as 9 per 1000 live births, making the United States rank 19th in infant mortality in the world.

T   F   2. The current recorded maternal mortality rate in the United States is approximately 8.3 per 100,000 live births.

T   F   3. The three major causes of maternal mortality are pregnancy-induced hypertension (PIH), hemorrhage, and pulmonary embolism.

T   F   4. Maternal mortality remains a significant problem because a high proportion of deaths are preventable.

T   F   5. The maternal mortality rate for African-American women is twice as high as that for Caucasian women.

T   F   6. African-American women are four times more likely than Caucasian women to give birth prematurely, have infants with low birth weight, and experience infant-fetal death.

T   F   7. Native-American mothers have the highest incidence of anemia, diabetes, pregnancy-associated hypertension, and uterine bleeding compared with all other racial or ethnic groups.

T   F   8. Respiratory distress syndrome continues as the leading cause of infant mortality during the first 4 weeks of life (the neonatal period).

T   F   9. The major outcome of antepartum testing is the detection of potential fetal compromise.

T   F   10. Serial measurement of the fetal biparietal diameter by means of ultrasonography may be helpful in estimating fetal age as well as growth.

T   F   11. Oligohydramnios or a decrease in amniotic fluid amount has been associated with neural tube defects, gastrointestinal obstructions, and multiple fetuses.

T   F   12. The presence of meconium in amniotic fluid antepartally is not usually associated with adverse fetal outcome.

T   F   13. After amniocentesis or chorionic villi sampling (CVS), an Rh-negative woman should receive RhoGAM.

T   F   14. The major disadvantage of a nonstress test relates to its high rate of false-negative results.

T   F   15. A lower than normal alpha-fetoprotein level in the maternal serum and in the amniotic fluid has been associated with Down syndrome.

T   F   16. To conduct a contraction stress test, four uterine contractions in a 15-min period are required.

T   F   17. A hyperstimulation result on a contraction stress test refers to late deceleration fetal heart rate (FHR) patterns, occurring as a result of excessive uterine activity or a persistent increase in uterine tone.

T   F   18. When performing a daily fetal movement count, a pregnant woman should call her health care provider if she notes eight or less fetal movements in 1 hr.

19. For each of the following categories, identify factors that would place the pregnant woman and her fetus/neonate at risk:

Biophysical

Psychosocial

Sociodemographic

Environmental

20. Regionalization of health care is a growing trend in the health care system of today.
    A. State the advantages of regionalization of maternal-newborn health care services.

    B. Indicate the purposes and goals for each of the following levels of facilities designated to provide maternity and neonatal care:
    Level I facilities

    Level II facilities

Level III facilities

21. Nonstress tests (NST) and contraction stress tests (CST) are antepartal diagnostic tests performed in the third trimester.
    A. State the rationale for performing these tests in the third trimester.

    B. List five indications for performing these tests.

    C. Indicate factors that are absolute contraindications for the performance of a contraction stress test.

22. Ally, a pregnant woman at 20 weeks gestation, is scheduled for a series of abdominal ultrasound tests to monitor the growth of her fetus. Describe the nursing role as it applies to Ally and ultrasound examinations.

23. State one risk factor for each of the following pregnancy problems:
    Preterm labor

    Polyhydramnios

Intrauterine growth restriction

Postterm pregnancy

Chromosomal abnormalities

Matching

Match the Antepartal Test in Column I with an indication for its use in Column II.

COLUMN I

A. Biophysical Profile
B. Daily Fetal Movement Count
C. Ultrasound
D. Cordocentesis
E. Amniocentesis
F. Chorionic Villi Sampling
G. Contraction Stress Test
H. Doppler Ultrasound
I. Triple Marker Test
J. Nonstress Test
K. Magnetic Resonance Imaging

COLUMN II

____ 24. Locate the placenta and grade its maturation.
____ 25. Estimate fetal maturity based on L/S ratio, presence of Pg, and levels of bilirubin, creatinine, and lipid cells.
____ 26. Evaluate five factors: FHR reactivity, fetal breathing movements, fetal body movements, fetal tone, and amniotic fluid volume.
____ 27. Measure blood flow and resistance in umbilical and uterine arteries.
____ 28. Screen for Down syndrome.
____ 29. Assess fetal well-being by maternal monitoring of fetal activity.
____ 30. Obtain fetal umbilical blood sample for prenatal diagnosis of health problems or perform an intrauterine transfusion.
____ 31. Determine FHR reaction to fetal activity.
____ 32. Assess for the presence of genetic abnormalities during the first trimester.
____ 33. Determine FHR response to uterine contractions.
____ 34. Evaluate maternal structures and biochemical status of tissues/organs.

Crossword Puzzle

Risk Assessment

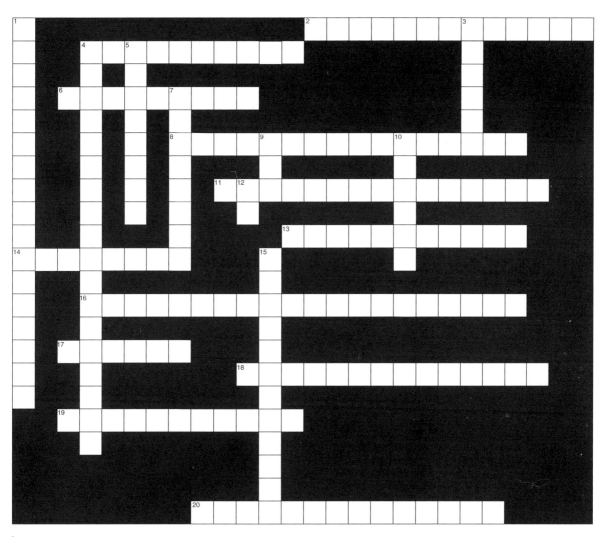

Across

2. Diagnostic test that involves the collection and examination of amniotic fluid.

4. Measurement of the _____ diameter after 12 wk gestation can assist in the estimation of gestational age and fetal growth.

6. _____ test is used to determine changes in the FHR pattern as a result of fetal movement.

8. An enzyme, if present at an elevated level in amniotic fluid or maternal serum, that can help to confirm the diagnosis of an open neural tube defect (i.e., spina bifida, anencephaly) or an open abdominal wall defect (omphalocele).

11. Diagnostic test that employs sound waves to examine structures. It can be used to assess the uterus and its contents, including the gestational sac, fetus, placenta, and amniotic fluid volume.

13. A _____ result to the NST is documented when no FHR acceleration, an acceleration of less than 15 BPM, or an acceleration lasting less than 15 sec occurs throughout any fetal movement during 40 min of the test.

14. A _____ result to the CST is documented when no late decelerations occur during a minimum of three uterine contractions lasting 40 to 60 sec within a 10-min period.

16. A phospholipid that, if present, reflects adequate fetal lung maturity. The incidence of respiratory distress syndrome is virtually 0%.

17. _____ test or titer is used to determine whether Rh antibodies are present in maternal serum.

18. Counting _____ on a daily basis by the pregnant woman can provide an indication of its well-being and facilitate the development of maternal-fetal attachment. (2 words)

19. The fetal _____ is present when fetal movements cease entirely for 12 hr. (2 words)

20. _____ sampling is a procedure done at 10 to 12 wk gestation. It involves the removal of a small tissue specimen from the fetal portion of the placenta for the purpose of genetic diagnosis. (2 words)

Down

1. A _____ test is used to determine the manner in which the FHR pattern will respond to a series of uterine contractions as may occur during labor. It determines the adequacy of uteroplacental circulation during a contraction. (2 words)

3. _____ simulation can be used as a method to release oxytocin from the posterior pituitary gland and thereby stimulate the contraction pattern required for a CST.

4. This is a noninvasive dynamic assessment of a fetus and its environment. The test employs sonography and external fetal monitoring. (2 words)

5. A _____ result to the CST is documented if persistent, consistent late decelerations occur with more than half of the contractions.

7. A _____ result to the NST is documented when two or more accelerations of the FHR of at least 15 BPM and lasting 15 sec or more occur in association with fetal movement over a 20-min period. A normal baseline range and long term variability of 10 BPM or more are also present.

9. The _____ test is used to differentiate maternal and fetal blood when vaginal bleeding occurs during pregnancy or labor.

10. Form of immune globulin that should be given to Rh-negative women following invasive diagnostic testing involving collection of amniotic fluid, fetal blood, or placental tissue.

12. A _____ ratio greater than 2:1 is one indicator of fetal lung maturity adequate for extrauterine survival.

15. A diagnostic test performed at 16 to 18 wk gestation that combines information from levels of maternal serum alpha-fetoprotein (MSAFP), unconjugated estriol, and human chorionic gonadotrophin (HCG). It is used to screen for the presence of Down syndrome.

Critical Thinking Exercises

1. Mary is at 42 weeks gestation. Her physician has ordered a biophysical profile (BPP). She is very upset and tells the nurse, "All my doctor told me is that this test will see if my baby is okay. I do not know what is going to happen and if it will be painful to me or harmful for my baby."
   A. Describe how the nurse should respond to Mary's concerns.

   B. Mary receives a score of 8 for the BPP. List the factors that were evaluated to obtain this score and specify the meaning of Mary's test result of 8.

2. Jan, age 42, is 18 weeks pregnant. Because of her age, Jan's fetus is at risk for genetic anomalies. Jan's blood type is A negative and her partner, the father of her baby, has B positive blood. Her primary health care provider has suggested an amniocentesis. Describe the nurse's role in terms of each of the following:
   A. Preparing Jan for the amniocentesis

   B. Supporting Jan during the procedure

   C. Providing Jan with post-procedure care and instructions

3. Susan, who has diabetes and is in week 36 of her pregnancy, has been scheduled for a nonstress test.

    A. Describe how you would prepare Susan for this test.

    B. Indicate how you would conduct the test.

    C. Analyze the following tracings. Designate the result each represents and indicate the criteria you used to determine the result.

      (1)

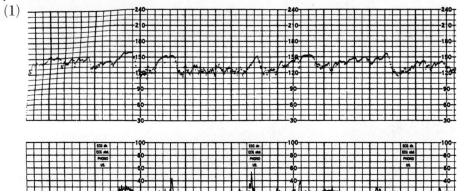

      (2)

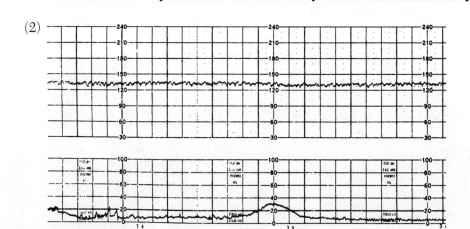

4. Beth arrives for a contraction stress test at the labor unit where you work. The physician has ordered that nipple stimulation be used to produce the required contractions.

   A. Describe how you would prepare Beth for the test.

   B. Indicate how you would conduct the test.

   C. Indicate how you would conduct the test differently if exogenous pitocin was used instead of nipple stimulation.

   D. Analyze the following tracings. Designate the result each represents and indicate the criteria you used to determine the results.

   (1)

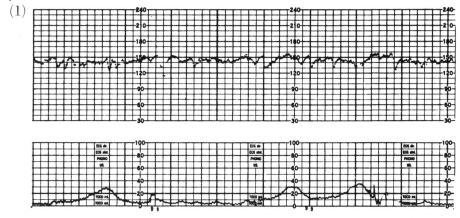

   (2)

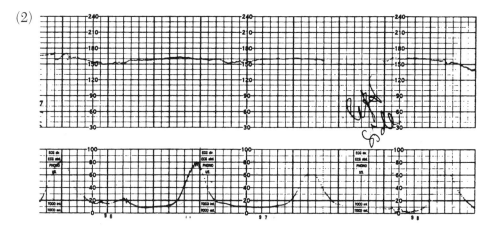

CHAPTER 23

Pregnancy at Risk: Preexisting Conditions

Chapter Review Activities

1. Describe the physiologic basis for the major signs and symptoms associated with diabetes mellitus.

   Hyperglycemia

   Polyuria

   Glycosuria

   Polydipsia

   Weight loss

   Polyphagia

Fill in the Blanks

2. Diabetes mellitus is a group of metabolic diseases characterized by _____ resulting from defects in _____, _____, or _____.

3. _____ refers to excretion of large volumes of urine. _____ refers to excessive thirst and _____ refers to excessive eating. Excretion of unusable glucose results in _____.

4. _____ is the label given to type 1 or type 2 diabetes that existed before pregnancy. _____ is any degree of glucose intolerance with onset of pregnancy or with first recognition occurring during pregnancy.

5. The key to optimal outcome of a diabetic woman's pregnancy is strict maternal _____ or _____ before and during pregnancy.

6. During the first trimester, insulin dosage for the patient with well-controlled diabetes may need to be reduced to avoid _____. There is an increased incidence of _____ episodes in women with type 1 diabetes during early pregnancy because _____, _____, and _____ result in dietary fluctuations, which influence maternal _____ levels and necessitate a reduction in insulin dosage.

7. During the second and third trimesters the dosage of insulin must be increased to avoid _____ and _____. _____ resistence begins as early as _____ and continues to rise until it stabilizes during the last few weeks of pregnancy.

8. For the pregnancy complicated by diabetes, fetal lung maturation is better predicted by the presence of _____ in the amniotic fluid rather than by the _____/_____ ratio.

9. Glycemic control over the previous 4 to 6 wk can be evaluated based on the determination of the level of _____ in the blood.

10. Dietary management during a diabetic patient's pregnancy must be based on _____ levels. Energy needs are usually estimated based on _____ cal/kg of ideal body weight. _____ of total calories should be from carbohydrates. _____ type carbohydrates should be limited, whereas _____ type carbohydrates should be emphasized when food choices are made. _____ of total calories should be from protein and less than _____ should be from fat.

11. Blood glucose levels are measured throughout each day: before _____, _____, and _____, and at _____. _____ measurements, 2 hr after meals may also be done. More frequent testing may be done during the _____ and _____ trimesters when insulin needs are _____.

12. Typically _____ of the daily insulin dose is given in the morning _____, using a combination of _____ and _____ insulin. The remaining _____ is administered in the evening _____. To reduce the risk of _____ during the night, often separate injections are given with _____ insulin given _____, followed by _____ insulin at _____.

13. Outline the major maternal and fetal/neonatal risks and complications associated with a diabetic patient's pregnancy.

   Maternal Risks/Complications   **Fetal and Neonatal Risks/Complications**

14. Complete the following table by identifying the metabolic changes that occur during pregnancy and indicating how these changes affect the woman with pregestational diabetes during the first trimester, the second and third trimesters, and the postpartum period.

Stage of Pregnancy	Metabolic Changes of Pregnancy	Impact on Diabetes
First trimester		
Second/Third trimesters		
Postpartum period		

15. State how hyperthyroidism and hypothyroidism can affect reproductive well-being and pregnancy.

True or False: Diabetes Mellitus During Pregnancy

Circle "T" if true or "F" if false for each of the following statements. Correct the false statements.

T   F   16. Insulin requirements may decrease during the first trimester but need to increase during the second and third trimesters.

T   F   17. Fasting blood glucose (FBS) levels should fall between 40 to 75 mg/dl.

T   F   18. Multiple injections of a mixture of NPH and regular insulin are usually required to maintain glucose control for the woman with pregestational diabetes, especially during the second half of pregnancy.

T   F   19. Ketoacidosis occurring at anytime during pregnancy can lead to intrauterine fetal death and is also a cause of preterm labor.

T   F   20. Congenital anomalies commonly associated with pregestational diabetes include limb deformities, malformations of the respiratory tract, and sensory deficits.

T   F   21. A glycosylated hemoglobin level of 13% to 20% indicates good glycemic control.

T   F   22. Diabetic women should avoid a bedtime snack when they are pregnant.

T   F   23. It is recommended that the 2 hr postprandial blood glucose level range be between 100 to 120 mg/dl.

T   F   24. As many as half of the women diagnosed with gestational diabetes may require insulin at some point during their pregnancy to maintain glycemic control.

T   F   25. The majority of women with gestational diabetes are asymptomatic during pregnancy.

T   F   26. Gestational diabetes is primarily a condition complicating the pregnancies of Caucasian women.

T   F   27. The incidence of congenital anomalies among infants of mothers with gestational diabetes is nearly the same as for infants of mothers with pregestational diabetes.

T   F   28. A 1-hr 50 gm glucose tolerance test result that is greater than 140 mg/dl indicates gestational diabetes.

T   F   29. Pregnant women with diabetes should test their urine in the morning and at bedtime to determine the presence of glucosuria, which would signal the onset of ketoacidosis.

T   F   30. To avoid the risk of fetal intrauterine death, labor should be induced as soon as the fetal lungs are mature, usually at approximately 36 weeks gestation.

T   F   31. Use of the tocolytics, ritodrine or terbutaline, to suppress preterm labor should be avoided with diabetic women because these medications increase the risk for hypoglycemia.

Crossword Puzzle

Health Problems Complicating Pregnancy (Hemorrhage, Hypertension, and Endocrine/Metabolic Disorders)

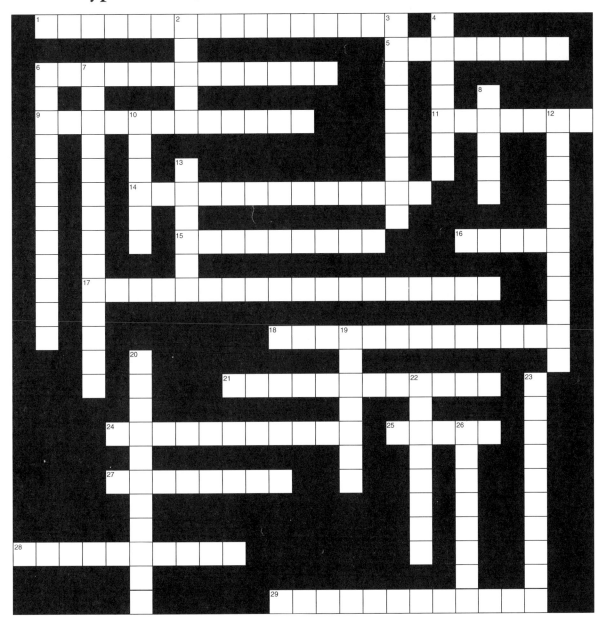

Across

1. _____ test measures the blood glucose level before and after administration of a 50 gm (1-hr test) or 100 gm (3-hr test) glucose load. (2 words)

5. Procedure whereby a band or ligature is placed around the cervix beneath the mucosa to constrict the internal os and thereby facilitate continuation of pregnancy to term.

6. _____ is documented as present when deep tendon reflexes are 3+ or greater.

9. A form of pregnancy-induced hypertension (PIH) characterized by hypertension, with protein-uria and/or generalized edema.

11. _____ pregnancy is one in which the fertilized ovum is implanted outside the uterine cavity, most often in the fallopian tube.

14. Diabetic state in which strict glycemic control is maintained and all parameters of fetal surveillance remain within normal limits is termed euglycemia or _____.

15. Arterial _____ has been identified as one of the underlying mechanisms for the signs and symptoms that occur with preeclampsia.

16. A syndrome experienced by severely preeclamptic women. It is characterized by destruction of red blood cells, liver involvement, and decreased platelet levels.

17. _____ restriction of the fetus occurs when placental perfusion is impaired as a result of health problems associated with pregnancy, such as PIH, diabetes, and cardiac dysfunction. (2 words)

18. A delay in the return of the uterus to normal size and function following pregnancy.

21. _____ hemoglobin is a test to measure glucose control over time by measuring the percentage of glucose-saturated hemoglobin in blood.

24. _____ diabetes refers to glucose intolerance first recognized during pregnancy, usually in the third trimester.

25. A _____ pregnancy is a type of gestational trophoblastic neoplasm that occurs as a result of a defective fertilization process.

27. Accumulation of blood in the soft tissues of the birth canal, including the vagina and perineum.

28. Increased fetal size with the infant weight above the 90th percentile. It is most often associated with maternal hyperglycemia and a resultant fetal hyperinsulinemia.

29. A state of hyperglycemia coupled with insulin deficiency that results in the mobilization of fatty acids.

Down

2. Generalized accumulation of fluid in the interstitial space after 12 hr of bedrest or a weight gain of >2 kg/wk. It is one of the signs characteristic of preeclampsia.

3. A form of pregnancy-induced hypertension (PIH) characterized by the occurrence of a convulsion and/or coma.

4. _____ is lost or spilled into the urine when perfusion of the kidneys is decreased as part of the pathophysiology involved with preeclampsia.

6. Low blood glucose that can occur in the pregnant diabetic woman, especially during the first trimester, and in newborns after birth.

7. _____ diabetic is the designation given to women with type 1 and type 2 diabetes who become pregnant.

8. Uterine _____ is marked hypotonia of the uterus that results in excessive bleeding and clotting after birth. It is the most common cause of postpartum hemorrhage.

10. Ankle _____ is documented as positive when rhythmic oscillations of one or more beats are felt when the foot is held in dorsiflexion and observed as the foot drops to the plantar flexed position.

12. _____ cervix, one cause of late spontaneous abortion and preterm birth, is characterized by painless dilatation of the cervical os without labor or uterine contractions, in the second or early third trimester of pregnancy.

13. Placenta _____ refers to implantation of the placenta in the lower uterine segment near or over the internal cervical os.

19. A combination of NPH and regular _____ is used to maintain glycemic control for women with pregestational diabetes.

20. _____ gravidarum is a condition that occurs when vomiting during pregnancy becomes excessive enough to cause weight loss as well as fluid, electrolyte, and acid-base imbalances.

22. Termination of pregnancy before viability of the fetus is achieved at about 20 to 24 weeks gestation, a fetal weight of greater than 500 gm, or a crown-rump length of 18 cm.

23. An excessive amount of amniotic fluid (>2000 ml). It is ten times more common in women with diabetes.

26. _____ placenta refers to premature separation of part or all of the placenta from its implantation site after the 20th week of pregnancy and before the birth of the baby.

True or False: Medical Problems Complicating Pregnancy

Circle "T" if true or "F" if false for each of the following statements. Correct the false statements.

T   F   32. Anemia is the most common medical disorder of pregnancy.

T   F   33. Folic acid anemia is the most common type of anemia in pregnancy.

T   F   34. Anemia predisposes the woman to postpartum infections.

T   F   35. Folic acid deficiency increases the incidence of neural tube defects, cleft lip, and cleft palate.

T   F   36. A well-balanced diet alone is unable to prevent iron deficiency anemia in pregnancy.

T   F   37. Oral iron supplementation should be taken in a dose of 60 mg three times a day beginning in the first trimester.

T   F   38. Exacerbations of sickle cell crises are diminished with pregnancy.

T   F   39. Preeclampsia, low birth weight, and fetal distress are more common in pregnancies complicated by thalassemia major.

T   F   40. Asthma increases the incidence of abortion and preterm labor.

T   F   41. Morphine should not be used to provide analgesia for laboring women with bronchial asthma because it may cause bronchospasm.

T   F   42. In pregnancy, adult respiratory distress syndrome (ARDS) is most likely to be precipitated by pulmonary embolism, disseminated intravascular coagulation (DIC), or aspiration pneumonia.

T   F   43. In the management of care for a laboring woman with cystic fibrosis, close monitoring of serum sodium and fluid balance is critical.

T   F   44. The pregnant woman is more vulnerable to cholecystitis than the nonpregnant woman.

T   F   45. More than 50% of women with rheumatoid arthritis experience a decrease in the severity of symptoms during pregnancy.

T   F   46. Infection is a leading cause of death among pregnant women with systemic lupus erythematosus (SLE).

T   F   47. Therapeutic abortion is recommended when a woman has multiple sclerosis, because pregnancy can cause irreversible worsening of the condition.

T   F   48. A pregnant woman with a cardiac problem may be experiencing cardiovascular decompensation if she notices a sudden inability to perform her usual activities as a result of fatigue and dyspnea.

T   F   49. Pregnant women with cardiac problems require a diet low in salt and potassium but high in easily digested, simple carbohydrates.

T   F   50. Women using heparin during pregnancy should increase their intake of foods high in vitamin K to enhance the anticoagulant effects of the drug.

T   F   51. Epidural anesthesia is more effective than narcotics for providing pain relief for a woman with cardiac problems who is in labor.

T   F   52. Internal monitoring should be avoided when assessing the FHR patterns of HIV-positive women during labor.

T   F   53. HIV can be transmitted to the newborn via the breast milk of an infected mother.

T   F   54. *Pneumocystis carinii* pneumonia is one of the opportunistic infections commonly seen in people with HIV and AIDS.

T   F   55. Zidovidine (AZT) should not be given to pregnant women who are HIV-positive, because it has been associated with fetal anomalies.

56. Identify the maternal and fetal complications most commonly seen in pregnant women with cardiac problems.

57. List the factors that can place a woman in the high risk category for HIV infection.

58. List the factors that increase the risk of perinatal HIV transmission.

True or False: Substance Abuse During Pregnancy

Circle "T" if true or "F" if false for each of the following statements. Correct the false statements.

T   F   59. It is estimated that substance abuse is a problem in over 25% of all pregnancies.

T   F   60. Every pregnant woman should be screened at least verbally for substance abuse at the first prenatal visit.

T   F   61. Meconium and hair of the newborn can be analyzed to determine the mother's past drug use over a longer period of time.

T   F   62. Disulfiram (Antabuse) is an effective substance to use during pregnancy for alcohol detoxification.

T   F   63. A woman dependent on a drug tends to exhibit a high degree of depression, with the abuse a way for women to blunt their feelings and relieve their psychologic distress.

T   F   64. Breastfeeding is safe for women who smoke marijuana.

T   F   65. Substance abusers often exhibit poor control over their behavior and a low threshold of pain during labor.

Critical Thinking Exercises

1. Mary is a 24-year-old diabetic woman. When Mary informed her gynecologist that she and her husband are trying to conceive a child, she was referred to an endocrinologist for preconception counseling. Mary tells the nurse that she cannot understand why this is necessary. "I have been a diabetic since I was 12 years old and I have not had many problems. All I want to do is get pregnant!" Discuss how the nurse should respond to Mary's comments.

2. Luann is a 25-year-old nulliparous woman in her first trimester of pregnancy (fourth week of gestation). She has had type 1 diabetes since she was 15 years old. Recently, she has been experiencing some nausea and is eating less as a result. She took her usual dose of regular and NPH insulin before eating a very light breakfast of tea and a piece of toast. Just before her midmorning snack at work she began to experience nervousness and tremors. She felt faint and became diaphoretic and pale.
   A. Identify the problem that Luann is experiencing. Indicate the basis for her symptoms.

   B. State the action that Luann should take.

3. Judy's pregnancy has just been confirmed. She also has type 1 diabetes.

   A. As a result of her high risk status a variety of additional assessment measures are emphasized during her prenatal period to evaluate the status of her fetus. Identify these additional assessment measures and their relevance in a diabetic pregnancy.

   B. Discuss the stressors that might confront Judy and her family as a result of her status as a diabetic woman who is pregnant.

   C. Complete the following table by describing the focus, nursing interventions, and health teaching for the major components of health care required at each stage of Judy's pregnancy.

Care Component	Antepartum	Intrapartum	Postpartum
Diet			
Glucose monitoring			
Insulin requirements			

   D. Indicate the activity and exercise recommendations that Judy should be given.

   E. After giving birth, Judy, who will be bottle feeding, asks the nurse about birth control. Discuss the birth control options that would be best for Judy and her partner.

4. Elena (2-1-0-0-1) is a 32-year-old Hispanic-American woman in week 28 of her pregnancy. She is obese. Her mother, who is 59 years old, was recently diagnosed with type 2 diabetes. Elena's first pregnancy resulted in the birth of a 10 lb, 6 oz daughter who is now 2 years old. A 1-hr, 50 gm glucose tolerance test last week revealed a glucose level of 152 mg/dl. A 3-hr glucose tolerance test was done yesterday with the following results: fasting, 108 mg/dl; 1 hr, 189 mg/dl; 2 hr, 170 mg/dl; 3 hr, 150 mg/dl.

A. Identify the complication of pregnancy Elena is exhibiting. State the rationale for your answer.

B. List the risk factors for this health problem that are present in Elena's assessment data.

C. Describe the pathophysiology involved in creating Elena's problem.

D. Identify the maternal and fetal/neonatal risks and complications possible in this situation.

E. Outline the ongoing assessment measures necessitated by Elena's health problem.

F. State the dietary changes Elena will have to make to maintain glycemic control during the rest of her pregnancy.

G. Before discharge after the birth of her second daughter, Elena asks the nurse if the health problem she experienced during this pregnancy will continue now that she has had her baby. She also wonders whether it will happen with her next pregnancy, because she wants to get pregnant again soon so she can "try for a son." Discuss the response the nurse should give to Elena's concerns.

5. Jennifer's pregnancy has just been confirmed. She has type 2 diabetes and is told that she now must learn how to give herself insulin. Jennifer became very upset and stated, "I cannot possibly give myself a shot. Why not let me continue to take my pills since they have been working fine so far?" Describe how you would respond to Jennifer.

6. Linda, age 26 years old, had rheumatic fever as a child and subsequently developed mitral valve stenosis. She is presently 6 weeks pregnant. This is the first pregnancy for Linda and her husband Sam. As part of her medical regimen, her primary health care provider substituted subcutaneous heparin for the oral warfarin sodium (Coumadin) she had been taking before pregnancy.

A. Linda states, "I cannot give myself a shot! Why can't I just take the medication orally?" Discuss how you would respond as to the purpose of heparin and why it must be used instead of Coumadin.

B. Indicate the information that the nurse should give Linda to ensure safe use of the heparin.

C. At 3 months gestation, Linda's cardiac condition is classified as class II according to the New York Heart Association's functional classification of organic heart disease. The classification, class II, means _____.
Discuss the therapeutic plan for this classification in terms of:
Rest/sleep/activity patterns

Prevention of infection

Nutrition

Bowel elimination

D. Identify physiologic and psychosocial factors that could increase the stress placed on Linda's heart during her pregnancy.

PHYSIOLOGIC FACTORS   **PSYCHOSOCIAL FACTORS**

E. List the symptoms that the nurse should teach Linda and her family to look for as indicators of possible cardiac decompensation.

F. List the objective signs that could indicate that Linda is experiencing signs of cardiac decompensation and heart failure.

G. Physiologic cardiac stress is greatest between _____ and _____ weeks gestation because _____.

H. Identify four nursing interventions related to the prevention of cardiac decompensation in Linda.

I. Linda is admitted to the labor unit. Her cardiac condition is still classified as class II. Outline the nursing measures designed to assess Linda and promote optimum cardiac function during labor and birth.

J. Linda should be observed carefully during the postpartum period, since her cardiac risk continues. The first _____ to _____ hours after birth will be the most hemodynamically difficult for Linda. Indicate the physiologic events after birth that place Linda at risk for cardiac decompensation.

K. Discuss the measures the nurse can use to reduce the stress placed on Linda's heart during the postpartum period.

L. Linda indicates that she wishes to breastfeed her infant. Describe the nurse's response.

M. Identify the important factors to be considered when preparing Linda's discharge plan.

7. Jean is a primigravida at 4 weeks gestation. She has been an epileptic for several years and her seizures have been controlled with phenytoin (Dilantin). Jean expresses concern regarding how her medication use will affect her pregnancy and her baby. She wants to stop taking the Dilantin. Describe the approach you would take in addressing Jean's concern and the course of action she is contemplating.

8. Martha is 4 weeks pregnant. As part of her prenatal assessment it was discovered that she was HIV positive.
   A. Specify nursing considerations related to enhancing Martha's health and well-being during each stage of her pregnancy.

   Prenatal stage

   Intrapartum stage

   Postpartum stage

   B. State the three modes of transmission of HIV from Martha to her fetus/newborn.

   C. Identify the measures that can be used to prevent transmission of HIV to Martha's baby.

9. Abuse of and dependence on psychoactive substances and alcohol have become pandemic.
   A. Discuss the approach the nurse should take during the first prenatal health history interview to screen a pregnant woman for alcohol and drug abuse.

   B. State the components of each of the following screening tests for alcohol abuse and explain how they are scored.

   T   **T**

   A   **W**

   C   **E**

   E   **A**

                                  K

   C. Identify the factors that the nurse should consider when planning care and setting expected outcomes for the pregnant woman who is dependent on psychoactive substance(s).

   D. Indicate the nursing measures appropriate for the woman who is dependent on drug(s) and alcohol during pregnancy, childbirth, and the postpartum period.

CHAPTER 24

Pregnancy at Risk: Gestational Conditions

Chapter Review Activities

1 Complete the following table by identifying the factors that distinguish the classifications of hypertensive disorders that can be present during pregnancy.

Hypertensive Disorder	Distinguishing Factors
Transient hypertension	
Preeclampsia	
Eclampsia	
HELLP syndrome	
Chronic hypertension	
Chronic hypertension with superimposed preeclampsia	

2. Contrast the expected physiologic adaptations of pregnancy with the ineffective responses to pregnancy characteristic of preeclampsia and eclampsia.

Expected Physiologic Adaptations   **Ineffective Responses**

3. State the principles you would follow to ensure the accuracy of blood pressure measurement during pregnancy.

True or False: Hypertension in Pregnancy

Circle "T" for true or "F" if false for each of the following statements. Correct the false statements.

T   F   4. Women with chronic renal disease or vascular disorders such as essential hypertension, diabetes mellitus, and lupus erythematosus are at increased risk for developing pregnancy-induced hypertension (PIH).

T   F   5. Low dose Tylenol is being investigated for the potentially beneficial effect it could have as a prophylactic treatment in the prevention of preeclampsia.

T   F   6. The increased incidence of preeclampsia and eclampsia in primigravidas and women pregnant by a new partner may be a result of immunologic responses.

T   F   7. When on bedrest, the woman with preeclampsia should maintain a dorsal recumbent position.

T   F   8. Sodium should be restricted to a minimal level when a woman has preeclampsia.

T   F   9. Women experiencing the HELLP syndrome often exhibit a platelet count of 400,000/mm^3 or higher.

T   F   10. Administration of magnesium sulfate to a woman with severe preeclampsia may precipitate labor by stimulating the uterus to contract.

T   F   11. An expected outcome for the use of magnesium sulfate is the prevention of progress from preeclampsia to eclampsia.

T   F   12. Hydralazine (Apresoline) may be used to lower the blood pressure of a woman with preeclampsia.

T   F   13. Epigastric or right upper-quadrant pain is a premonitory symptom of impending eclampsia.

T   F   14. A diet that is low in protein and fat but high in calcium is recommended to women with preeclampsia.

T   F   15. Prompt treatment of a woman using appropriate medications, bedrest, and diet can cure preeclampsia.

T   F   16. Methergine is the oxytocic of choice to prevent or treat postpartum hemorrhage for women with preeclampsia.

17. List the risk factors associated with the development of PIH.

18. Describe the assessment technique used to determine if the following findings are present in women with preeclampsia. Note: you may wish to review this information in a physical assessment textbook for a complete explanation of each technique.
    Hyperreflexia

    Ankle clonus

    Proteinuria

    Pitting edema

19. Preeclampsia affects fetal well being.
    A. Describe how preeclampsia can adversely affect the health and well being of the fetus.

    B. Indicate the fetal surveillance measures recommended for women experiencing preeclampsia.

Matching

Match the client description in Column I with the appropriate diagnosis from Column II.

COLUMN I

_____ 20. At 30 weeks gestation, Angela's MAP ranged from 108 mm Hg to 114 mm Hg. Urinalysis indicated protein content of +2; a weight gain of 2 kg in one week and upper body edema were noted.

_____ 21. At 24 weeks gestation, Mary's BP was noted to have risen to 148/92 from a prepregnant baseline of 110/66. No other problematic signs and symptoms were noted.

_____ 22. Susan, a 34-year-old pregnant woman, has been noted to have a consistently high BP ranging from 148/92 to 160/98 since she was 28 years old. Her weight gain has followed normal patterns and urinalysis remains normal as well.

_____ 23. At 32 weeks gestation, Maria, with hypertension since 28 weeks and exhibiting generalized edema and proteinuria of +3, has a convulsion.

_____ 24. Dawn has been hypertensive since her 24th week of pregnancy. Urinalysis indicates a protein content of +3. Further testing reveals a platelet count of 95,000 mm^3 and elevated AST and ALt levels; in addition, burr cells appear on a peripheral smear.

COLUMN II

A. Eclampsia
B. Chronic hypertension
C. Transient hypertension
D. HELLP Syndrome
E. Preeclampsia

25. Identify three measures to prevent preeclampsia that are currently being researched for effectiveness.

True or False: Hemorrhagic Complications During Pregnancy

Circle "T" if true or "F" if false for each of the following statements. Correct the false statements.

T   F   26. Spontaneous abortions are often related to maternal behavior.

T   F   27. There is little that nurses can do to reduce the incidence of early or late spontaneous abortions.

T   F   28. A missed abortion refers to a pregnancy in which the fetus has died but spontaneous abortion does not occur.

T   F   29. An etiologic factor for incompetent cervix is use of diethylstilbestrol by the woman's mother during pregnancy.

T   F   30. The most common site for an ectopic pregnancy is the ampulla of the uterine tube. Ectopic pregnancies account for 10% of all maternal deaths.

T   F   31. Ectopic pregnancy is the leading pregnancy-related cause of second trimester maternal mortality.

T   F   32. Ectopic pregnancy is a leading cause of infertility.

T   F   33. Infertile women who use Clomid to stimulate ovulation are at higher risk for development of hydatidiform mole.

T   F   34. Previous cesarean birth, multiple gestation, and closely spaced pregnancies increase the risk for placenta previa.

T   F   35. A vaginal examination performed when a woman is exhibiting signs of placenta previa can result in profound hemorrhage.

T   F   36. A blood-saturated peri-pad weighing 200 gm would reflect a 300 ml blood loss.

T   F   37. Premature separation of the placenta accounts for 15% of all perinatal deaths, and about one third of infants born to mothers with premature separation of the placenta die.

T   F   38. Abdominal trauma is a major risk factor for abruptio placentae.

Fill in the Blanks

Insert the appropriate term for bleeding during pregnancy for each description.

39. Early in pregnancy _____, _____, _____, or _____ is the most common causes for excessive bleeding.

40. Late in pregnancy _____, _____, or _____ may cause hemorrhage.

41. _____ is defined as the termination of pregnancy that occurs before the fetus is able to _____. In the United States this period is before _____ weeks of gestation. A fetal weight of less than _____ may also be used to define this type of pregnancy loss. There are five types of this form of pregnancy termination, namely _____, _____, _____, _____, and _____.

42. Evaluation of the serum level of the placental hormone _____ and assessment of the viability of the _____ using _____ are two diagnostic tests that can be used when a pregnant woman is exhibiting signs of threatened abortion.

43. Placenta previa is described as total or complete if the _____ is _____ covered by the placenta when the cervix is fully dilated; as partial if the _____ is _____ covered; and as marginal if only an _____ of the placenta extends to the _____. Risk for postpartum hemorrhage is increased because the _____ is unable to _____ around the open blood vessels of the placental site.

44. _____ or abruptio placentae is the _____ of _____ or _____ of the placenta from its _____ site. A woman who experienced abruptio placentae is at higher risk for postpartum hemorrhage as a result of _____ and/or _____.

45. Disseminated intravascular coagulation (DIC) can result from a number of obstetric problems.
A. Identify three predisposing conditions for DIC.

B. Describe the pathophysiology that leads to DIC.

C. Indicate the clinical manifestations of DIC that would be noted during physical examination and with laboratory testing.

D. Describe four priority nursing measures that should be used when caring for a woman experiencing DIC.

Matching

Match the diagnosis in Column I with the appropriate diagnosis in Column II.

COLUMN I

_____ 46. Placental anomaly in which the cord vessels begin to branch at the membranes and then course out at the placenta.

_____ 47. Fertilized ovum is implanted outside the uterine cavity.

_____ 48. Termination of pregnancy before fetal viability as a result of natural causes.

_____ 49. Complication of abruptio placentae that occurs when blood accumulates between the placenta and the uterine wall thereby reducing uterine contractility.

_____ 50. Placental implantation in the lower uterine segment.

_____ 51. Painless dilatation of the cervical os without uterine contractions, often resulting in an inability to carry the pregnancy to term.

_____ 52. Fertilization of an ovum whose nucleus has been lost or inactivated resulting in the formation of a mass of fluid-filled vesicles that resemble a bunch of white grapes.

_____ 53. Premature separation of part or all of the placenta from its implantation site.

_____ 54. Cord insertion at the margin of the placenta.

_____ 55. Placenta is divided into two or more separate lobes.

COLUMN II

A. Incompetent cervix
B. Abruptio placentae
C. Hydatidiform mole (complete)
D. Battledore placenta
E. Ectopic pregnancy
F. Succenturiate placenta
G. Placenta previa
H. Spontaneous abortion
I. Couvelaire uterus
J. Velamentous cord insertion

56. Trauma continues to be a common complication during pregnancy that may require obstetric critical care.
    A. Discuss the significance of this complication using statistical data to describe the scope of the problem in terms of incidence, timing during pregnancy, and forms of trauma.

    B. Indicate the effects trauma can have on pregnancy.

    C. Describe the potential effect of trauma on the fetus.

    D. Explain why the nurse must be alert for signs and symptoms of abruptio placentae for at least 48 hours after the trauma occurred.

57. Priorities of care for the pregnant woman following trauma must be to _____ and _____. This method of approach in care management is important since _____ survival is dependent on _____ survival. In cases of minor trauma the woman is evaluated for vaginal _____, uterine _____, abdominal _____, _____, or _____, and evidence of _____. A change in or absence of _____ or _____, leakage of _____, and presence of _____ in maternal circulation are also included in the assessment. In cases of major trauma, the systematic evaluation begins with a _____ and the initial "ABCs" of resuscitation: _____, _____, and _____.

58. Complete the following table by identifying each priority activity for perinatal trauma management and the responsibilities of the team caring for the mother and the team caring for the fetus.

Priority Activity	Maternal Team	Fetal Team
T		
R		
A		
U		
M		
A		

59. Complete the following table by identifying recommended treatment measures and nursing considerations for each infection.

Infection	Treatment Measures	Nursing Considerations
Bacterial vaginosis		
Candidiasis		
Chlamydia		

Infection	Treatment Measures	Nursing Considerations
Gonorrhea		
Group B *Streptococcus*		
Hepatitis B		
Herpes		
Human papillomavirus		
Syphilis		
Trichomonas		

Fill in the Blanks: TORCH Infections

Insert the appropriate term for TORCH infections for each of the following descriptions.

60. A viral infection of the liver that is transmitted by droplets or hands washed improperly after defecation.

_____

61. Three-day German measles that can produce major congenital anomalies during the first trimester and systemic and intrauterine growth restriction (IUGR) after the fourth month.

_____

62. A protozoan infection transmitted by consumption of infected raw or undercooked meat or with poor handwashing after handling infected cat litter.

_____

63. A viral infection transmitted via contact with body secretions/fluids including respiratory, genitourinary, breast milk, and blood. Fetal infection can cause mental retardation, microcephaly, and eye, ear, and dental defects.

_____

64. A viral infection of the liver transmitted in a manner similar to HIV.

_____

65. A viral infection transmitted primarily by sexual contact. Active infection of the genital tract at the time of labor often requires cesarean birth.

_____

66. A viral infection of the liver commonly found in IV substance abusers and recipients of multiple blood transfusions. There is no immunoprophylaxis yet available.

_____

Critical Thinking Exercises

1. Jean (2 - 1 - 0 - 0 - 1) is at 30 weeks gestation and has been diagnosed with mild preeclampsia. The treatment plan includes home care with bedrest with bathroom privileges and out of bed twice a day for meals, appropriate nutrition, and stress reduction. She and her husband are very anxious about the diagnosis and are also concerned about how they will manage the care of their active 3-year-old daughter Anne.

   A. Indicate the signs and symptoms that would have been present to indicate this diagnosis.

   B. List three priority nursing diagnoses for Jean and her family.

   C. Describe how you would help this couple to organize their home care routine.

   D. Specify what you would teach them with regard to assessment of Jean's status as well as signs of worsening preeclampsia.

   E. Describe the instructions you would give Jean regarding her nutrient and fluid intake.

   F. Discuss the measures Jean can use to cope with the bedrest requirement of her treatment plan.

2. Ellen, a pregnant woman at 37 weeks gestation, is admitted to the hospital with a diagnosis of severe preeclampsia.

   A. Indicate the signs and symptoms that would have been present to indicate this diagnosis.

   B. List three prioriy nursing diagnoses for Ellen.

   C. Specify the precautionary measures that should be taken to protect Ellen and her fetus from injury.

   D. Ellen's physician orders magnesium sulfate to be infused at 4 gm in 20 minutes as a loading dose then a maintenance intravenous infusion of 2 gm/hr.

      (1) Identify the guidelines that must be followed when administering magnesium sulfate IV piggyback.

      (2) Explain the expected therapeutic effect of magnesium sulfate to Ellen and her family.

      (3) List the maternal-fetal assessments that should be accomplished on a regular basis during the infusion of magnesium sulfate.

(4) Identify the signs of magnesium sulfate toxicity.

(5) State the interventions that must be instituted immediately if magnesium sulfate toxicity occurs.

E. Despite all prevention efforts, Ellen has a convulsion.
   (1) Specify the nursing measures that should be implemented at the onset of the convulsion and immediately afterward.

   (2) List the problems that can occur as a result of the convulsion that Ellen experienced.

F. Ellen successfully gave birth vaginally despite her high-risk status. Describe Ellen's care management during the first 48 hours of her postpartum recovery period.

3. Marie, an 18-year-old primigravida, is diagnosed with hyperemesis gravidarum. She is admitted to the high-risk antepartal unit.
   A. Identify the predisposing and etiologic factors related to Marie's health problem.

   B. List the physiologic and psychosocial factors the nurse should be alert for when assessing Marie.

C. State two priority nursing diagnoses related to Marie's health problem.

D. Outline the nursing care measures appropriate for Marie.

4. At times pregnant women require abdominal surgery.
   A. Identify the factors that can complicate diagnosis of and surgical treatment for abdominal problems during pregnancy.

   B. Identify three common conditions that necessitate abdominal surgery during pregnancy.

   C. Preoperative care for a pregnant woman differs from that for a nonpregnant woman in one significant aspect, namely the presence of the _____. General preoperative observations and ongoing care are the same as for any surgery, with the addition of continuous _____ and _____ monitoring. Intraoperatively, fetal oxygenation is improved by placing the woman on an operative table with a _____ to avoid maternal _____. Continuous _____ and _____ monitoring must take place during the surgical procedure and in the postoperative period if intrauterine pregnancy continues.

   D. Identify the nursing considerations and topics for teaching related to the discharge planning process of the pregnant woman who experienced abdominal surgery.

5. Andrea is admitted to the hospital where she is diagnosed as having an acute ruptured ectopic pregnancy in her fallopian tube.
   A. State the risk factors associated with ectopic pregnancy.

B. Describe the findings most likely experienced and exhibited by Andrea as her ectopic pregnancy progressed and then ruptured.

C. Identify the other health-care problems that share the same or similar clinical manifestations as ectopic pregnancy.

D. The major care management problem in ectopic pregnancy when the tube ruptures is _____.

E. _____ therapy is being explored as a nonsurgical treatment approach for women with a very early (<6 weeks) ectopic pregancy. This therapy causes _____ of the ectopic pregnancy.

F. Identify two priority nursing diagnoses appropriate for Andrea.

G. Outline the nursing measures required during the preoperative and postoperative periods.

6. Janet is 10 weeks pregnant. She comes to the clinic and states that she has been experiencing slight bleeding with mild cramping for about 4 hours. No tissue has been passed, and pelvic examination reveals that the cervical os is closed. Her fundal height is consistent with a 10 week pregnancy.

A. Indicate the most likely basis for Janet's signs and symptoms.

B. Outline the expected care management of Janet's problem.

7. Denise, a primigravida, calls the clinic. She is crying while she tells the nurse that she has noted "a lot of bleeding" and that she is sure she is losing her baby.

   A. Identify the questions the nurse should ask Denise in order to obtain a more definitive picture of the bleeding she is experiencing.

   B. Based on the data collected, Denise is admitted to the hospital for further evaluation. Her signs and symptoms progress, and medical diagnosis of incomplete abortion is made. Describe the assessment findings that would indicate the diagnosis of incomplete abortion.

   C. State the nursing diagnosis that would take priority at this time.

   D. Outline the nursing measures that would be appropriate for the priority nursing diagnosis you identified and for the expected medical management of Denise's health problem.

   E. Specify the instructions that Denise should receive before her discharge from the hospital.

   F. List the nursing measures appropriate for the nursing diagnosis: anticipatory grieving related to unexpected outcome of pregnancy.

8. Mary has been diagnosed with hydatidiform mole (complete).
   A. Identify the typical signs and symptoms Mary would most likely exhibit to establish this diagnosis.

   B. Specify the post treatment instructions that the nurse must stress when discussing follow-up management with Mary.

   C. A major concern associated with hydatidiform mole is the development of _____, which is indicated by a rising _____ titer and enlarging _____.

9. Two pregnant women are admitted to the labor unit with vaginal bleeding. Sara is at 29 weeks gestation and is diagnosed with marginal placenta previa. Jane is at 34 weeks gestation and is diagnosed with a moderate (grade II) premature separation of the placenta (abruptio placentae).
   A. Compare the clinical picture each of these women is likely to exhibit during assessment.
   SARA   **JANE**

   B. Contrast the care management approach required for each of the women as it relates to their diagnosis and the typical medical management.
   SARA   **JANE**

   C. Indicate the considerations that must be given top priority following birth for each of these women.
   SARA   **JANE**

CHAPTER 25

Labor and Birth at Risk

Chapter Review Activities

1. State the criteria used to diagnose each of the following abnormal labor patterns:
   A. Prolonged latent phase

   B. Protracted active phase

   C. Secondary arrest

   D. Protracted descent

   E. Arrest of descent

F. Failure of descent

G. Precipitous labor

2. Describe each of the five factors that cause labor to be long, difficult, or abnormal. Explain how they interrelate.

3. Angela is experiencing hypertonic uterine dysfunction, Bernice is experiencing hypotonic uterine dysfunction, and Gloria is having difficulty bearing down effectively. Contrast each woman's labor in terms of causes/precipitating factors, maternal-fetal effects, change in pattern of progress, and care management.

	Angela (Hypertonic)	Bernice (Hypotonic)	Gloria (Inadequate Expulsion)
Causes/ precipitating factors			
Maternal-fetal effects			
Change in pattern of progress			
Care management			

4. Postterm or postdate birth is the birth of an infant beyond the end of week _____ of gestation or _____ days from the first day of the last menstrual period (LMP). It is found to occur in an average of _____ of births. The most common cause of postdate pregnancy is _____ because the woman had an _____ pattern. Deficiency of placental _____ may also be a cause. A major concern is the effect on the fetus of placental _____, a process that begins after _____ weeks gestation. Another concern is the decrease in amniotic fluid volume resulting in _____ and which can lead to _____ of the umbilical cord.

5. Identify maternal risks inherent in postdate pregnancy and birth.

6. Identify the fetal/neonatal risks inherent in postdate pregnancy, labor, and birth.

7. Outline the typical care management measures for postdate pregnancy.

8. Specify the instructions that the nurse should give to a woman experiencing a postdate pregnancy.

Membranes can rupture at anytime during pregnancy and childbirth.
9. Premature rupture of membranes is the rupture of the _____ before _____ begins. It occurs in approximately _____ of all pregnancies and is the most common cause of preterm labor. At term uterine contractions begin in most women within _____ hours after rupture, but labor may not start for up to _____ after rupture of membranes in women between 28 to 34 weeks gestation. If membranes rupture before 38 weeks gestation, it is called _____. If membranes are ruptured for more than 24 hours before birth, it is called _____. The cause of premature rupture of membranes is _____ in most instances. Premature rupture of membranes can result in _____ and _____, and in _____ and _____ of the umbilical cord as a result of _____ and _____. _____ of amniotic fluid from the cervix using a sterile speculum examination, a positive _____ test result, or the presence of _____ by dried amniotic fluid on a slide are all signs of ruptured membranes.

10. List the factors that are typically associated with premature rupture of membranes.

11. Specify the instructions that a woman should be given who has experienced premature rupture of membranes and is discharged to home care.

Matching

Match the description in Column I with the appropriate term in Column II.

COLUMN I

_____ 12. Stimulation of uterine contractions after the spontaneous onset of labor yet progress is unsatisfactory

_____ 13. Primary dysfunctional labor usually occurring during the latent phase

_____ 14. Ineffective primary or secondary powers preventing progress of cervical dilatation and/or fetal descent

_____ 15. A period of 4 to 6 hours of spontaneous, active labor to determine if vaginal birth is safe for maternal-fetal unit

_____ 16. Long, difficult, or abnormal labor caused by problems associated with the five essential factors of labor

_____ 17. A labor that lasts < 3 hours from onset of contractions to the time of birth

_____ 18. Slowing or arrest of labor progress in terms of dilatation and/or descent

_____ 19. Initiation of contractions before their spontaneous onset to bring about birth

_____ 20. Secondary uterine inertia usually occurring during the active phase

COLUMN II

A. Dystocia
B. Hypotonic uterine dysfunction
C. Precipitous labor
D. Trial of labor
E. Dysfunctional labor
F. Augmentation of labor
G. Abnormal labor patterns
H. Induction of labor
I. Hypertonic uterine dysfunction

Preterm labor and birth create significant risks for the newborn.

21. Preterm birth occurs after the _____ week but before the end of the _____ week of gestation. Categories of risk factors implicated in preterm birth include _____, _____, and _____. In approximately half of preterm births the cause is _____. The incidence of preterm birth in the United States is approximately _____. Preterm birth is responsible for almost _____ of infant deaths. _____ agents are drugs that inhibit uterine contractions. An antidote for ritodrine and terbutaline is _____ and an antidote for magnesium sulfate is _____. _____ is a glucocorticoid that can reduce the incidence of respiratory distress syndrome in preterm infants less than _____ weeks gestation when given at least _____ hours before birth. While on bedrest during preterm labor suppression, the woman should maintain a _____ position to optimize _____ and decrease pressure on the _____.

22. Identify specific etiologic factors for each risk category that increase the vulnerability of women to the onset of preterm labor and birth.

23. Discuss the health-care and lifestyle measures you would encourage a woman at risk for preterm labor to adopt as a means of preventing its onset.

24. Identify the signs of preterm labor that you would teach to pregnant women, especially those at increased risk.

25. Describe the actions a woman should take if she is at home and begins to notice early signs of preterm labor such as a contracting uterus.

26. Outline the protocol a nurse should follow when a woman is admitted to the labor unit with a diagnosis of preterm labor.

27. State the maternal and fetal side effects of ritodrine/terbutaline.

28. State the maternal side effects of magnesium sulfate.

29. Discuss the controversy of bedrest as a component of the care management of women who experience high-risk pregnancies including preterm labor.

Amniotic fluid embolism (AFE) is a serious, potentially life-threatening complication of pregnancy.

30. An amniotic fluid embolism occurs when _____ containing _____ enters the maternal _____ and obstructs _____ causing _____ and _____. This complication is estimated to be associated with a maternal mortality rate as high as _____ and a fetal mortality rate of _____. Maternal death occurs most often if _____ is present in the fluid because it _____ the pulmonary vessels more completely than other debris. Serious coagulation problems such as _____ usually occur. _____ is an additional problem that often accompanies amniotic fluid embolism. Maternal factors such as _____, tumultuous _____, _____, and _____, and fetal problems such as _____, _____, and _____ have been associated with an increased risk for development of amniotic fluid embolism.

31. List the signs of amniotic fluid embolism for each of the following categories:
    A. Respiratory distress

    B. Circulatory collapse

    C. Hemorrhage

32. Outline the recommended care management of a woman experiencing an amniotic fluid embolism.

33. Identify four indications for oxytocin induction and four contraindications to the use of oxytocin to stimulate the onset of labor.
    A. Indications

    B. Contraindications

Crossword Puzzle

Labor and Birth at Risk

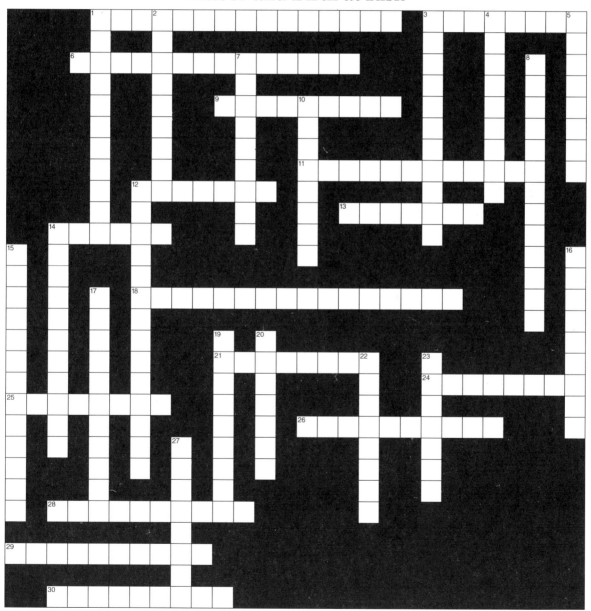

Across

1. Administration of effective analgesics to reduce pain and encourage sleep for women experiencing primary dysfunctional labor. (two words)

3. _____ birth is the birth of an infant beyond the end of the 42nd week of gestation or 294 days from the first day of the last menstrual period.

6. Hormones that can be applied to the cervix in order to make it softer and thinner.

9. Initiation of uterine contractions before their spontaneous onset for the purpose of bringing about birth.

11. Stimulation of uterine contractions after labor has started spontaneously yet progress is unsatisfactory.

12. Procedure whereby the fetus is turned artificially from one presentation to another. It may be accomplished internally or externally.

13. _____ of descent is a lack of descent of the presenting part during the deceleration phase and the second stage of labor.

14. The most common malpresentation of the fetus, with the buttocks presenting first through the pelvis.

18. Alternative medication to the sympathomimetics used for the suppression of labor with fewer side effects. (two words)

21. An _____ active phase of the first stage of labor is diagnosed when either a nulliparous or a multiparous woman demonstrates no progress for more than 2 hours.

24. Hormone produced by the pituitary gland that stimulates uterine contractions.

25. _____ of the umbilical cord occurs when the cord lies below the presenting part of the fetus. Compression of the cord can result.

26. A _____ active phase of the first stage of labor is diagnosed when the cervix dilates at a rate of less than 1.2 cm/hr for the nullipara and less than 1.5 cm/hr for the multipara.

28. Pregnancy with a gestation of two or more fetuses.

29. _____ uterine dysfunction or primary dysfunctional labor is often associated with an anxious nulliparous woman experiencing painful uterine contractions out of proportion to the intensity or effectiveness of the contractions.

30. A _____ latent phase of the first stage of labor is one that exceeds 20 hours in the nullipara or 14 hours in the multipara.

Down

1. Preferred sympathomimetic drug to suppress preterm labor. A subcutaneous pump system can be used to allow for home care of the woman experiencing preterm labor.

2. The first and only sympathomimetic drug approved by the FDA to inhibit preterm labor. The cardiovascular system is most affected in terms of side effects.

3. A _____ labor is defined as a labor that lasts less than 3 hours from the onset of contractions.

4. _____ medications are a classification of drugs that inhibit uterine contractions.

5. An amniotic fluid _____ occurs when amniotic fluid containing particles of debris enters the maternal circulation and obstructs pulmonary vessels causing respiratory distress and circulatory collapse.

7. Procedure used to artificially rupture the membranes.

8. _____ labor is described as abnormal uterine contractions that prevent normal progression of cervical effacement, dilatation, and/or ineffective maternal bearing down efforts, interfering with fetal descent.

10. _____ birth is the birth of the fetus through a transabdominal incision of the uterus.

12. A _____ birth is the application of a special cup to the fetal head and use of negative pressure to facilitate birth. (two words)

14. A rating system used to determine cervical ripeness and its inducibility or ability to respond to stimulation of labor. (two words)

15. _____ disproportion results in an inability of the fetal head to fit through the maternal pelvis in order to be born vaginally.

16. _____ uterine dysfunction or secondary uterine inertia is associated with a slowing of progress during the active phase of the first stage of labor.

17. A beta-blocking agent used as an antidote when serious side effects occur as a result of using beta-adrenergic agents (sympathomimetics) to suppress labor.

19. _____ tents can be used as a mechanical method of thinning and softening the cervix.

20. _____ labor is the onset of regular uterine contractions that cause cervical changes between 20 and 37 weeks of gestation.

22. A long, difficult, or abnormal labor caused by various conditions associated with the five factors of labor.

23. Instruments with two curved blades used to assist in the birth of the fetal head.

27. Process of softening and thinning of the cervix that can occur naturally or as a result of using chemical or mechanical agents.

Critical Thinking Exercises

1. Denise, a primigravida, has reached the second stage of her labor with her fetus at zero station and positioned left occipitoposteriorly. She is experiencing intense low back pain. Denise did not attend any childbirth classes and is having difficulty pushing effectively. No anesthesia has been used.
   A. Identify the factors that can have a negative effect on the secondary powers of labor (bearing down efforts).

   B. Describe how you would help Denise to use her expulsive forces to facilitate the descent and birth of her baby.

   C. Specify the positions that would be recommended based on the position of the presenting part of Denise's fetus.

2. Anne, a primigravida, attended Lamaze classes with her husband, Mark. They were looking forward to working together during the labor and birth of their baby. Because of fetal distress, an emergency low segment cesarean section with a transverse incision was performed after 18 hours of labor. Even though Anne and her son are in stable condition, she expresses a sense of failure because, "I could not manage to give birth to my son in the normal way and now I never will!"
   A. List the preoperative nursing measures that should have been implemented to prepare Anne physically and emotionally for the unexpected cesarean birth.

B. Specify the assessment measures that are critical when Anne is in the recovery room following her birth.

C. State the postoperative nursing care measures that Anne requires.

D. Just before discharge Anne asks the nurse if there is any chance a vaginal birth will be possible if she gets pregnant again. Describe how the nurse should respond to Anne's question.

3. A vaginal examination reveals that Marie's fetus is in a right sacroanterior position. Specify the considerations that the nurse should keep in mind when providing care for Marie.

4. Angela is at 42 weeks gestation and has been admitted for induction of her labor.
   A. Assessment of Angela at admission included determination of her Bishop's Score. State the purpose of the Bishop's Score and identify the factors that are evaluated.

   B. Angela's score was 5. Interpret this result in terms of the planned induction of her labor.

   C. Angela's primary health-care provider ordered that Cervidil be inserted. State the purpose of the Cervidil, method of application, and potential side effects that can occur.

D. Before inducing her labor, Angela's primary health provider performs an amniotomy. Specify the nursing responsibilities before, during, and after this procedure.

E. Indicate which of the following actions reflect appropriate care (A) for Angela during the induction of her labor with intravenous oxytocin. If the action is not appropriate (NA) state what the correct action would be.

(1) _____ Apply an external electronic fetal monitor and obtain a 15 to 20 minute baseline strip of fetal heart rate and pattern.

(2) _____ Explain to Angela what to expect and techniques used.

(3) _____ Prepare a primary line with an isotonic electrolyte solution.

(4) _____ Attach the secondary line of dilute oxytocin (10U in 1000 ml) to the distal port (farthest from the venipuncture site) of the primary IV.

(5) _____ Begin infusion at 4 mU/min.

(6) _____ Increase oxytocin by 1 to 2 mU/min at 5- to 10-minute intervals after the initial dose until the desired pattern of contractions is achieved.

(7) _____ Stop increasing the dosage when contractions occur every 2 to 3 minutes, last 40 to 90 seconds, and reach an intrauterine pressure between 40 to 80 mm Hg if internal monitoring is being used.

(8) _____ Administer meperidine (analgesic) intravenously to Angela through the secondary line containing the oxytocin.

(9) _____ Monitor maternal blood pressure and pulse every 15 minutes.

(10) _____ Monitor fetal heart rate pattern and uterine activity every 15 minutes.

(11) _____ Limit IV intake to 1500 ml/8 hr.

F. State the major side effects of pitocin for which the nurse must be alert when managing Angela's labor.

G. List the nursing actions to be taken if hyperstimulation of the uterus occurs.

5. Debra has been experiencing signs of preterm labor. After a period of hospitalization, her labor was successfully suppressed and she was discharged to be cared for at home. Debra is receiving terbutaline via a subcutaneous pump. She will record her uterine activity twice a day with an ambulatory tokodynamometer device. Debra must also remain on bedrest.
   A. Outline what you would teach Debra regarding the care and maintenance of the terbutaline subcutaneous pump that is being used.

   B. Identify the side effects of terbutaline that the nurse should teach Debra before discharge.

   C. Describe the instructions that Debra should be given regarding home uterine monitoring.

   D. Debra has two children who are 5 and 8 years old. Specify the suggestions you would give to help Debra and her children cope with the bedrest requirement ordered by Debra's primary health-care provider.

CHAPTER 26

Postpartum Complications

Chapter Review Activities

Fill in the Blanks: Physical Complications Related to Childbirth

Insert the term that corresponds to each of the following descriptions:

1. _____ is the loss of more that 1,000 ml of blood. Additional criteria that may be used are a decrease in _____ of 10 or more percentage points or a need for _____ therapy. The leading cause is _____.

2. Marked hypotonia of the uterus is called _____.

3. A _____ is the accumulation of blood in tissue as a result of blood vessel damage. It is usually associated with a forceps-assisted birth, performance of an episiotomy, or being a primigravida. The woman often complains of persistent _____ or _____ pain or a feeling of pressure in the _____.

4. _____ refers to the turning of the uterus inside out. The primary signs of its presence are _____, _____, and _____. Contributing factors include _____ pressure, _____ applied to the umbilical cord, _____, _____, and an abnormally adherent _____.

5. _____ is the delayed return of the enlarged puerperal corpus to normal size and function.

6. _____ is an emergency situation in which profuse blood loss (hemorrhage) can result in severely compromised perfusion of body organs. Death may occur.

7. A _____ is suspected when bleeding is continuous and there is no identifiable cause. _____ is an autoimmune disorder in which antiplatelet antibodies decrease the lifespan of the platelets. _____ is a type of hemophilia and is probably the most common of all hereditary bleeding disorders.

8. A _____ is the formation of a blood clot or clots inside a blood vessel and is caused by _____ or partial _____ of the vessel. _____ involves the superficial saphenous venous system. For _____ involvement varies but can extend from the foot to the iliofemoral region. _____ occurs when part of a blood clot dislodges and is carried to the pulmonary artery, where it occludes the vessel and obstructs blood flow to the lungs.

9. _____ refers to any clinical infection of the genital canal that occurs within 28 days after abortion or childbirth. The first symptom is usually a _____ of 38° C or more on _____. Common infection sites are _____, _____, _____, _____, and _____.

10. _____ or _____ infection is the most common cause of postpartum infection. It usually begins at the _____ site.
11. _____ is an infection of the breast affecting approximately 1% of women, soon after childbirth, most of whom are _____.
12. _____ is a variation of the normal placement of the uterus, the most common type of which is _____ or retroversion.
13. Downward displacement of the uterus is known as _____. This dropping down of the uterus can range from mild to complete.
14. _____ is a protrusion of the bladder downward into the vagina. It develops when supporting structures in the vesicovaginal septum are injured.
15. _____ is the herniation of the anterior rectal wall through the relaxed or ruptured vaginal fascia and rectovaginal septum.
16. Uncontrollable leakage of urine is known as _____. When it occurs as a result of sudden increases in intraabdominal pressure associated with sneezing, coughing, or laughing it is called _____.
17. A _____ is an abnormal communication (opening) between one hollow viscus (organ) and another, or from one hollow viscus to the outside. A communication between the bladder and the genital tract is called a _____ and one between the rectum and the vaginal tract is called a _____.
18. A _____ is a device that can be placed in the vagina to support the uterus and hold it in the correct position.
19. Surgical repair of a cystocele is called _____ whereas _____ is the surgical repair of a rectocele.

True or False

Circle "T" if true or "F" if false for each of the following statements. Correct the false statements.

T   F   20. Early postpartum hemorrhage usually occurs as a result of uterine atony.

T   F   21. When a woman hemorrhages, changes in her baseline vital sign values may not be reliable indicators of shock in the immediate postpartum period because of the physiologic adaptations that occurred during pregnancy.

T   F   22. Dark red blood is a characteristic finding when deep lacerations of the cervix bleed.

T   F   23. Methergine is the oxytocic of choice for postpartum hemorrhage if the woman is also experiencing preeclampsia.

T   F   24. Prostaglandin $F_2\alpha$ (Hemabate) should be used with caution or not at all if the postpartum woman has asthma.

T   F   25. Subinvolution of the uterus is the second major cause of early postpartum hemorrhage.

T   F   26. For most women, the placenta separates within 30 minutes of childbirth.

T   F   27. Placenta accreta refers to a placenta that perforates the uterus.

T   F   28. Uterine inversion occurs most frequently in primiparous women with abruptio placenta.

T   F   29. The woman with third- or fourth-degree laceration should not be given rectal suppositories or enemas to facilitate bowel elimination.

T　F　30. Administration of blood and blood components can lead to hyperthermia, bradycardia, and metabolic alkalosis.

T　F　31. Aspirin or aspirin-containing analgesics can be safely used if a woman is receiving heparin because aspirin enhances its effect.

T　F　32. The most effective and cheapest treatment method for postpartum infection is prevention.

T　F　33. Mastitis usually develops in the second to fourth week postpartum.

T　F　34. Lactation must be suppressed once mastitis is diagnosed.

T　F　35. The most common type of uterine displacement is retroversion.

T　F　36. Symptoms of pelvic relaxation most often appear during the perimenopausal period as a result of decreasing ovarian hormone secretion.

T　F　37. Good hygiene of the genital area is critical when a pessary is being used.

T　F　38. An anterior and posterior colporrhaphy is a surgical procedure performed to repair a uterine prolapse.

39. List the factors that would increase the risk for each of the following complications associated with childbirth:

A. Lacerations of the birth canal

B. Hematomas of the birth canal

C. Retained placenta

D. Inversion of the uterus

E. Subinvolution of the uterus

40. Hemorrhagic shock is an obstetric emergency. List the signs and symptoms indicative of hemorrhagic shock.

41. State the two-fold focus of medical management of hemorrhagic shock.

42. Identify four priority nursing interventions for hemorrhagic shock.

43. State the standard of care for bleeding emergencies.

44. Identify effective measures to prevent genital tract infections that the nurse should teach postpartum women.

True or False: Postpartum Depression and Mood Disorders

Circle "T" if true or "F" if false for each of the following statements. Correct the false statements.

T   F   45. Female babies are especially vulnerable to the effects of poorer cognitive outcome when a postpartum mood disorder results in the disruption of the mother-infant interaction.

T   F   46. Mothers with low self-esteem are more likely to experience postpartum depression than mothers with high self-esteem.

T   F   47. Women who feel close to their husbands report fewer depressive symptoms.

T   F   48. A postpartum mood disorder with psychotic features occurs in 1 or 2 women per 1,000 live births.

T   F   49. Once a woman has had a postpartum episode with psychotic features, there is little risk it will occur again with a subsequent pregnancy.

T   F   50. Women with postpartum depression may experience suicidal ideation and obsessional thoughts regarding violence to their newborns.

T   F   51. Women with postpartum depression are rarely treated with antidepressant medications.

Postpartum psychologic complications have major implications for the mother, her newborn, and entire family.

52. The definition of postpartum depression without psychotic features is an _____ and _____ with _____ and _____. The incidence is from _____ to _____ of new mothers. These symptoms rarely disappear without outside help. A distinguishing feature of postpartum depression is _____. A prominent finding of postpartum depression is _____ of the infant often caused by abnormal _____.

53. State the predisposing factors for postpartum depression.

54. List the clinical manifestations that must be present nearly every day to diagnose a major depression.

55. A common nursing diagnosis for postpartum depression would be altered parent-infant attachment related to limited ability of the mother to interact with and care for her infant, secondary to postpartum depression. Identify the nursing measures appropriate for this nursing diagnosis.

56. Cite measures and activities that can be used to prevent postpartum depression.

57. Postpartum psychosis is a syndrome most often characterized by _____, _____, and thoughts by the mother of _____. Symptoms of this syndrome often begin within _____ after birth, although the mean time to onset is _____ and almost always within _____ of the birth. Characteristically, the woman begins to complain of _____, _____, and _____ and may have episodes of _____ and _____. Later, _____, _____, _____, _____, and _____ about the baby's well-being may be present. Delusions, when present, often are related to the _____ and in severe cases auditory hallucinations may command the mother to _____. A specific illness included in depression with psychotic features is _____ formerly called manic-depressive illness. This mood disorder is preceded or accompanied by _____ episodes and is characterized by _____, _____, or _____ moods.

58. State the focuses for care management of the woman with postpartum depression with psychotic features as they relate to the woman herself, her baby, and her family.

Critical Thinking Exercises

1. Postpartum hemorrhage (PPH) is a leading cause of maternal mortality.
   A. An early, acute primary postpartum hemorrhage occurs within the _____ after birth. A late or secondary postpartum hemorrhage occurs more than _____ after birth but less than _____ postpartum. The most common cause of postpartum hemorrhage is _____.
   B. Contrast the causative factors for early postpartum hemorrhage with the causative factors for late postpartum hemorrhage.

   Early postpartum hemorrhage

   Late postpartum hemorrhage

   C. Identify the most common risk factors for uterine atony.

   D. The initial management of excessive postpartum bleeding is _____ with _____, elimination of any _____ and _____. If the uterus fails to respond then a _____ dose of _____ or _____ may be given _____ or _____ to produce sustained _____. If first line drugs are ineffective then a derivative of _____ may be given _____.
   E. Outline the noninvasive assessments of cardiac output that should be performed on a frequent and ongoing basis in postpartum patients who are bleeding.

F. Identify three nursing diagnoses associated with postpartum hemorrhage.

G. List, in order of use, the oxytocics that function to stimulate uterine contraction when atony is present. Indicate the usual administration routes, dosage, and specific contraindications/precautions for each medication listed.

2. Nurses working on a postpartum unit must be constantly alert for signs and symptoms of puerperal infection in their clients.
   A. List the factors that can predispose postpartum women to puerperal infection.

   B. Identify the infection prevention measures that should be used when caring for pregnant and postpartum women.

   C. State the typical signs and symptoms of endometritis.

   D. Describe the critical nursing interventions.

3. Sara, a breastfeeding mother at 2 weeks postpartum, begins to exhibit signs and symptoms of mastitis.
   A. List the typical signs and symptoms of mastitis.

   B. Identify the measures that could have been used to prevent the occurrence of mastitis.

   C. Describe the treatment measures and health teaching that Sara needs regarding her infection and breastfeeding, since she wishes to continue to breastfeed.

4. Teresa (6-5-0-1-5), a 60-year-old postmenopausal woman, has been diagnosed with a moderate uterine prolapse, accompanied by cystocele and rectocele.
   A. Describe the signs and symptoms Teresa most likely exhibited for this diagnosis to have been established.

   B. Outline the nursing care management approach recommended for Teresa's health problem.

   C. Teresa will use a pessary during the day until a surgical repair can be accomplished. Specify the instructions you would give to Teresa regarding the use and care of a pessary.

5. Mary, a 35-year-old primiparous woman, is bottle feeding her infant and is beginning her second postpartum week. She and her husband Tom moved from Buffalo, where they lived all their lives, to Los Angeles 2 months ago to take advantage of a career opportunity for Tom. They live in a community with many other young couples who are also starting families. Last month they joined the Catholic church near their home. Tom tries to help Mary with the baby, but he has to spend long hours at work to establish his position. When making a home visit as part of an early discharge program, the nurse identifies that Mary is exhibiting behaviors strongly suggestive of postpartum depression. Mary is concerned that she is not being a very good mother and stating "I just do not know what to do sometimes and I am not even breastfeeding."

   A. Identify the predisposing factors for postpartum depression that are present in Mary's situation.

   B. Indicate the signs and symptoms Mary most likely exhibited to lead the nurse to come to this conclusion.

   C. Specify several questions that the nurse could ask Mary to determine the depth of postpartum depression that she is experiencing.

   D. Describe the measures the nurse could use to help Mary and Tom cope with postpartum depression.

CHAPTER 27

The Newborn at Risk: Problems Related to Gestational Age

Chapter Review Activities

Fill in the Blanks

Insert the appropriate term for each description.

1. An infant born before completion of 37 weeks' gestation, regardless of birth weight is termed _____.

2. An infant born between the beginning of week 38 and the end of week 42 of gestation is termed _____.

3. An infant who is born after the completion of week 42 of gestation is termed

   _____.

4. An infant born after 42 weeks of gestation who exhibits the effects of progressive placental insufficiency is termed _____.

5. An infant whose weight is above the 90th percentile for gestational age is termed

   _____.

6. An infant whose weight falls between the 10th and the 90th percentiles for gestational age is termed _____.

7. An infant whose weight is below the 10th percentile for gestational age is termed

   _____.

8. The fetus whose rate of growth does not meet expected norms is said to have

   _____.

9. An infant whose birth weight is 2,500 gm or less is termed _____. These infants are considered to have had either _____ or _____. _____ and _____ commonly occur together.

10. An infant whose birth weight is 1,500 gm or less at birth is termed _____.

11. Infants weighing more than _____ and born after _____ of pregnancy have the best prospect for survival.

12. Preterm birth is responsible for almost _____ of the infant deaths.

13. There is a dramatic reduction in mortality in infants regardless of weight who are born after _____.

14. The preterm infant is at risk because of _____ and _____.

15. List the common causes/risk factors for each of the following:
    Preterm birth

    Large for gestational age newborns

    Small for gestational age newborns

    Intrauterine growth restriction

16. Explain the purpose of exogenous surfactant administration to the preterm newborn.

17. The preterm infant is vulnerable to a number of complications related to immaturity of body systems. Complete the following table by identifying the potential problems and the physiologic basis for each physiologic function listed.

Physiologic Function	Potential Problems	Physiologic Basis
Respiratory Function		
Cardiovascular Function		
Maintaining Body Temperature		
Central Nervous System Function		
Maintaining Adequate Nutrition		
Maintaining Renal Function		
Maintaining Hematologic Status		
Resisting Infection		

True or False

Circle "T" if true or "F" if false for each of the following statements. Correct the false statements.

T F 18. Examination of the anterior vascular capsule of the lens of infants less than 27 weeks gestation will reveal corneas that are too hazy for the lens vessels to be visualized.

T F 19. Eight months after birth, an infant born at 30 weeks gestation would be considered to be the corrected age of $5\frac{1}{2}$ months.

T F 20. The incidence of physical and emotional abuse is slightly higher toward the infant who, because of preterm birth or illness, was separated from the mother for a period of time after birth.

T F 21. Sudden infant death syndrome (SIDS) is three to four times more prevalent among preterm infants as compared with term infants.

T F 22. Neonatal respiratory distress with hypoxemia can result in closure of the ductus arteriosus.

T F 23. Many large-for-gestational-age newborns are born well after the estimated date of birth.

T F 24. Not all postdate infants are postmature.

T F 25. Hypoglycemia is defined as a blood glucose level of less than 50 mg/dl in both term and preterm infants during the first 3 days of life.

T F 26. Fetal hypoglycemia stimulates peristalsis in the intestine resulting in a passage of meconium.

T F 27. Acrocyanosis is an assessment finding indicative of an underlying respiratory disorder.

T F 28. The flow rate for a gavage tube feeding should approximate that of an oral feeding (1 ml/min).

T F 29. Compromised infants usually have lower caloric, nutrient, and fluid requirements than those of the full-term, normal newborn.

T F 30. A decrease in rectal temperature is often an early sign of cold stress in the newborn.

T F 31. Compromised infants often require an oxygen saturation greater than 95% to maintain respiratory stability because their hemoglobin levels are often low.

T F 32. Infants born before 36 weeks gestation require exogenous surfactant administration to survive extrauterine life.

T F 33. Infants who need oxygen should have their respiratory status assessed accurately every 1 to 2 hours.

34. Explain kangaroo care.

35. When providing care, nurses need to consider the pain experienced by newborns, especially those who are compromised and require numerous invasive procedures.
    A. Describe pain assessment according to each of the following categories:
       Behavioral responses

Physiologic/autonomic responses

Metabolic responses

B. Discuss how each of the following strategies can be used to manage the pain experienced by newborns:

Nonpharmacologic management

Pharmacologic management

36. Respiratory distress syndrome (RDS) is a lung disorder usually associated with preterm birth.
    A. The pathophysiology of respiratory distress syndrome is due to a lack of _____ that leads to progressive _____, loss of _____, and a _____ imbalance, with uneven distribution of _____.
    B. Clinical signs of respiratory distress syndrome include _____, _____, _____, _____, _____ increasing work of _____, _____, _____ or _____ acidosis, and _____ and _____. These symptoms usually appear immediately after _____ or within _____. Physical examination reveals _____, _____, _____, use of _____, and occasionally _____.
    C. RDS is usually self-limiting with respiratory symptoms abating after _____ hours. The disappearance of symptoms coincides with _____ production.
    D. Treatment of respiratory distress syndrome involves establishment and maintenance of adequate _____ and _____, administration _____, and maintenance of a _____ environment.

Matching: Complications Associated with Oxygen Therapy

Match the description in Column I with the appropriate term in Column II.

COLUMN I

_____ 37. Disorder of developing blood vessels in the eye often associated with oxygen tensions that are too high for the level of retinal maturity, initially resulting in vasoconstriction and continuing problems after the oxygen is discontinued.

_____ 38. Acute inflammatory disease of the gastrointestinal mucosa that is commonly complicated by perforation.

_____ 39. Disorder related to insufficient surfactant production.

_____ 40. Occurs when fetal shunt between the pulmonary artery and the aorta fails to constrict after birth or reopens after constriction has occurred.

_____ 41. Chronic pulmonary condition in infants who have experienced respiratory failure, oxygen dependence for longer than 28 days and continued beyond 36 weeks' postconceptual age, abnormal radiographic findings with areas of overinflation and areas of atelectasis, and respiratory symptoms.

_____ 42. One of the most common types of brain injury encountered in the neonatal period and among the most severe in both short-term and long-term outcomes.

COLUMN II

A. Respiratory distress syndrome (RDS)

B. Bronchopulmonary dysplasia (BPD)

C. Retinopathy of prematurity (ROP)

D. Patent ductus arteriosus (PDA)

E. Periventricular-intraventricular hemorrhage (PV-IVH)

F. Necrotizing enterocolitis (NEC)

Critical Thinking Exercises

1. Oxygen therapy is a vital component in the care of the newborn experiencing respiratory distress.

   A. Identify the criteria that should be used to determine if there is a need for supplemental oxygen.

   B. Create a set of general guidelines that reflects the recommended principles for safe and effective administration of oxygen to a compromised newborn.

C. Complete the following table by specifying the indications for each of the following methods of oxygen therapy and describing the care measures required to ensure their safe and effective administration.

Method	Indications	Nursing Measures
Hood		
Nasal Cannula		
Continuous Positive Airway Pressure		
Mechanical Ventilation		

2. The goal of weaning is the withdrawal of all oxygen support.
   A. Describe signs indicative of an infant's readiness to be weaned from oxygen therapy.

   B. Outline the guidelines that should be followed when weaning a newborn from oxygen therapy.

3. Anne is a 3 pound, 12 ounce (1,705 gm) preterm newborn at 32 weeks gestation and is admitted to the neonatal intensive care nursery (NICU) after her birth for observation and supportive care. Anne's nutritional needs are a critical concern in her care. Oral formula feedings are attempted first.

A. State the assessment data that the nurse should document after each of Anne's feedings to indicate feeding method effectiveness.

B. The acceptable weight loss limit during Anne's first week of life is _____ of her birth weight. After the first week, Anne's loss or gain during each 24-hour period should not exceed _____ of the previous day's weight. Possible causes for weight loss include _____, _____, _____, or _____, and _____.

C. The nurse determines that Anne's suck is weak and she becomes too fatigued during oral feedings to obtain sufficient nutrients and fluid. The nurse confers with the neonatologist and a decision is made to provide intermittent gavage feedings with occasional oral feedings. Describe the procedure the nurse should follow when inserting the gavage tube.

D. State the priority nursing diagnosis for Anne.

E. Discuss the principles the nurse should follow before, during, and after a gavage feeding to ensure safety and maximum effectiveness.

F. Outline the protocol that should be followed when advancing Anne back to full oral feeding.

4. The NICU is a stressful environment for preterm infants and their families.
   A. Identify the common sources of stress facing infants and their families in an intensive care environment.

   Infant Stressors   **Family Stressors**

   B. Nurses working in the ICN must be aware of infant cues and adjust stimuli accordingly. List infant cues that indicate overstimulation and infant cues that indicate a relaxed state.

   Overstimulation

   Relaxed State

   C. Identify specific measures that can be used to protect infants from overstimulation and yet provide appropriate stimulation to meet their developmental and emotional needs.

   D. Specify the guidelines that should be followed regarding infant positioning.

   E. Describe the measures a nurse can use to help the parents and family cope with their infant's death.

5. Mary and Jim are parents of a preterm baby boy.
   A. Parental responses to their preterm newborn progress through several stages. Match Mary and Jim's comments and behaviors in Column I with the appropriate stage in Column II.

   COLUMN I
   _____ 1. Mary says to Jim, "Did you see him yawning?"
   _____ 2. Jim is excited, "Did you see how he smiled at me?"
   _____ 3. Jim asks the nurse, "What is his temperature today?"
   _____ 4. Mary changes her baby's diaper after feeding him.
   _____ 5. Mary looks at her baby's face while stroking and touching him.
   _____ 6. Mary and Jim tell the nurse that they named their baby James because he "looks just like his dad as a baby."

   COLUMN II
   A. Stage one
   B. Stage two
   C. Stage three

   B. State the parental tasks that need to be accomplished by Mary and Jim, as parents of a preterm infant.

   C. Describe the nursing measures that should be used to support Mary and Jim and facilitate their progress through the stages and tasks of parenting a preterm infant.

6. Marion's pregnancy appears to be entering week 43.
   A. Support this statement: Perinatal mortality is significantly higher in the postmature fetus and neonate.

   B. State the assessment findings that are typical of a postmature infant.

   C. Identify the potential complications experienced by a postmature infant.

7. Janet, a pregnant woman at term, is in labor. On the basis of serial ultrasound findings, her fetus is estimated to be smaller that it should be as a consequence of Janet's heavy smoking during pregnancy and her high-risk status related to preeclampsia. Identify the four major complications facing Janet's baby during labor, birth, and the postpartum period. Describe the physiologic basis for each potential complication and the signs and symptoms indicative of its presence.

CHAPTER 28

The Newborn at Risk: Acquired and Congenital Conditions

Chapter Review Activities

True or False: Hyperbilirubinemia and Congenital Disorders

Circle "T" if true or "F" if false for each of the following statements. Correct the false statements.

T F 1. When physiologic jaundice is experienced by Caucasian and African-American infants the level of unconjugated bilirubin in the serum peaks at a higher level than in Asian or Native-American infants and takes one week or longer to resolve.

T F 2. A cephalhematoma, hemangioma, or ecchymosis can increase the newborn's risk for hyperbilirubinemia.

T F 3. For the full-term infant a serum bilirubin of 15 mg/dl is considered the upper limit at which the risk for kernicterus increases.

T F 4. Kernicterus usually appears within 24 to 48 hours following birth.

T F 5. The most common causes of pathologic hyperbilirubinemia are hemolytic disorders in the newborn (HDN).

T F 6. ABO incompatibility is more common that Rh incompatibility but causes less severe problems in the affected infant.

T F 7. At birth an indirect Coombs' test is performed on the newborn's cord blood to determine if the fetus has produced antibodies to its mother's blood.

T F 8. Major congenital disorders are the leading cause of death among infants younger than 1 year of age in the United States.

T F 9. Certain congenital heart defects (CHD) may not become apparent until the infant or child exhibits symptoms when exposed to stressors such as growth demands or infection.

T F 10. The causes for congenital heart defects are readily identified in almost all cases.

T F 11. Closure of spina bifida cystica is usually delayed until the infant is approximately 6 months of age.

T F 12. An infant with a left-sided diaphragmatic hernia should be positioned on its left side, with its head and chest elevated.

T F 13. Clubfoot occurs more frequently in females than in males.

14. Describe the physiologic basis for ABO incompatibility.

15. Specify the events that can result in a woman developing antibodies to the Rh factor, a process called _____ or _____.

16. Congenital anomalies affect the health and well-being of infants.
    A. A disease or disorder that is transmitted from generation to generation is termed _____ or _____. A _____ disorder is one that is present at birth and can be caused by _____ or _____ factors, or both. Many defects appear to occur as a result of _____ inheritance, which is the interaction of _____, with _____ factors that affect development. Examples of these include _____, _____, _____, and _____ or _____. The most common major congenital anomalies that cause serious problems for the neonate are _____, _____, _____, or _____, _____, and _____.

    B. Specify the assessment techniques and considerations that guide perinatal diagnosis of congenital anomalies.

    C. Explain why observation of the amount of amniotic fluid can be helpful in the perinatal diagnosis of certain congenital anomalies.

    D. Indicate how each of the following types of postnatal tests can be used to diagnose an infant with a congenital anomaly:
    Biochemical tests

    Cytological studies

    Dermatoglyphics

17. Congenital heart defects (CHDs) are a major cause of death in the first year of life.
    A. List the maternal factors that are associated with a higher incidence of CHDs.

    B. Identify the four physiologic categories of CHDs and give one example for each category.

    C. Describe the signs that may be exhibited at birth by an infant with a CHD.

18. Name the congenital disorder represented by each of the following descriptions:
    A. A group of recessive gene disorders that results from an absence of or a change in a protein, usually an enzyme. Examples include phenylketonuria and galactosemia. _____
    B. A small brain is present in a normally formed head. _____.
    C. The urinary meatus opens below the glans penis or anywhere along the ventral surface of the penis, scrotum, or peritoneum. _____ When the urethral opening is on the dorsal surface of the penis, it is called _____.
    D. Enlargement of the ventricles of the brain, usually as a result of interference with the circulation and absorption of cerebrospinal fluid. It is characterized by a bulging anterior fontanel, an abnormal increase in the circumference of the head, and an increasing intracranial pressure. _____
    E. Ventricular septal defects and tetralogy of Fallot are two common forms of this type of congenital disorder. _____
    F. The most common form of clubfoot. The foot points downward and inward, the ankle is inverted, the Achilles tendon is shortened. _____
    G. A common congenital anomaly of the nose requiring emergency surgery after birth. It consists of a bony or membranous septum between the nose and the pharynx. _____
    H. A form of spina bifida cystica (a neural tube defect) in which an external sac containing the meninges and spinal fluid protrudes through a defect in the vertebral column.
       _____
    I. A covered defect of the umbilical ring into which varying amounts of the abdominal organs may herniate. It is covered with a peritoneal sac. _____
    J. The passageway from the mouth to the stomach ends in a blind pouch or narrows into a thin cord, thus a continuous passageway to the stomach is not present. _____
    K. A type of central nervous system anomaly characterized by the absence of both cerebral hemispheres and the overlying skull. It is incompatible with life. _____
    L. Disorder characterized by displacement of the abdominal organs into the thoracic cavity.
       _____
    M. A form of spina bifida cystica (a neural tube defect) in which an external sac containing the meninges, spinal fluid, and nerves protrudes through a defect in the vertebral column.
       _____

19. Birth injuries, although decreasing in incidence, are still an important source of neonatal morbidity.

   A. Identify the factors that increase fetal vulnerability to injury and trauma at birth.

   B. Describe the signs indicative of a fractured clavicle and the usual approach to treatment.

True or False: Birth Trauma and the Effects of Maternal Infection and Substance Abuse

Circle "T" if true or "F" if false for each of the following statements. Correct the false statements.

T F 20. The Apgar Score can alert nurses to the possibility that a birth injury occurred and identify infant need for immediate resuscitation.

T F 21. Birth injuries are a very minor source of neonatal morbidity.

T F 22. Subconjunctival hemorrhage present at birth requires immediate treatment to prevent permanent ocular damage.

T F 23. The presentation of the fetus can affect the type and location of birth injuries.

T F 24. Petechiae and ecchymosis will not blanch when digital pressure is applied.

T F 25. Fracture of the femur during the birth process is the most common birth injury.

T F 26. Neonatal spinal cord injuries are almost always a result of a difficult birth from the breech presentation.

T F 27. Although the mother infected with toxoplasmosis (a protozoan infection) often exhibits no signs and symptoms, she has a 90% chance of transmitting the infection to her fetus.

T F 28. The primary mode of transmission of gonorrhea to the fetus or newborn is via an infected birth canal.

T F 29. Maternal infection with syphilis is most dangerous during the first trimester as organogenesis takes place.

T F 30. Penicillin is the antibiotic choice for treating syphilis.

T F 31. Even with adequate treatment, the neonate infected with syphilis may experience complications as late as 15 years of age.

T F 32. Major teratogenic effects of rubella involve the cardiovascular system, the ears, and the eyes.

T F 33. The infant infected with the rubella virus may be a serious source of infection to susceptible individuals, particularly women in their childbearing years.

T F 34. Newborns infected with cytomegalovirus must begin receiving penicillin therapy within 24 hours of birth.

T F 35. Snuffles is a common assessment finding exhibited by infants infected with herpes simplex virus.

T F 36. A primary maternal infection with the herpes simplex virus after 32 weeks gestation presents a greater risk to the fetus or newborn than a recurrent herpes simplex virus infection.

T   F   37. The most common cause of neonatal sepsis and meningitis in the United States is group B *Streptococcus.*

T   F   38. Hepatitis B during pregnancy is associated with an increased risk for malformations, stillbirths, and intrauterine growth restriction.

T   F   39. In order to prevent a chlamydial infection of the eyes, silver nitrate should be instilled over the cornea of the newborn's eyes immediately after birth.

T   F   40. Infants born to mothers who drank socially during pregnancy may exhibit fetal alcohol effect, which could include learning, speech, and behavioral problems.

T   F   41. Maternal heroin use results in a high rate of congenital anomalies.

T   F   42. Marijuana use during pregnancy may result in shortened gestation and a higher incidence of intrauterine growth restriction (IUGR).

Fill in the Blanks: Diabetes in Pregnancy and Effect on the Neonate

43. As a result of stricter control of _____ and improved _____, there has been a(n) _____ in perinatal mortality in diabetic pregnancy. The incidence of congenital anomalies is still _____ than the general population. During early pregnancy, congenital anomalies are caused by fluctuations in _____ and episodes of _____. Later in pregnancy, maternal _____ forces high levels of _____ to cross the placenta, stimulating the fetal pancreas to secrete increased amounts of _____. This event results in excessive fetal _____ termed _____. In addition, if the blood of a pregnant diabetic woman becomes more _____ than fetal blood, _____ or _____ exchange will be diminished. There are indications that some neonatal conditions, namely _____, _____, _____, _____, and perhaps fetal _____ may be eliminated or the incidence decreased if maternal _____ levels are maintained within narrow limits.

44. Identify the most common congenital anomalies experienced by infants with diabetic mothers in terms of each of the following:
Cardiac

Central nervous system

Musculoskeletal

45. Baby boy Robert, weighing 11 pounds 4 ounces, was born 1 hour ago. His mother has pregestational diabetes.

A. Describe the typical characteristics exhibited by a macrosomic infant such as Robert.

B. The macrosomic infant is most at risk for the complications of _____, _____, _____, and _____.

C. Describe the warning signs of potential complications of which the nurse should be aware when assessing Robert during the first 24 hours after his birth.

D. State the infections(s) represented by each letter in the acronym TORCH.

T

O

R

C

H

46. Sepsis is one of the most significant causes of neonatal morbidity and mortality.
   A. Complete the following table by identifying the modes for infection transmission during each of the periods below and indicating the major sites of infection.

Period	Mode of Transmission	Infection Sites
Prenatal		
Perinatal		
Postnatal		

   B. Identify the risk factors that, if present, should alert the nurse to the increased potential for infection in the neonate.

   C. List the signs a neonate might exhibit that would indicate that sepsis is present.

   D. Describe two effective nursing measures for each of the following categories.
   Prevention   **Cure**   **Rehabilitation**

Critical Thinking Exercises

1. Pathologic jaundice or hyperbilirubinemia is a serious health problem with the potential for severe complications that can permanently affect the life and health of the infant.
   A. Describe how time of onset and resolution along with serum levels of unconjugated bilirubin can be used to differentiate physiologic jaundice from the more serious pathologic jaundice.

B. The yellowish discoloration of the skin, mucous membranes, sclera, and other organs is called _____. The deposit of bilirubin in the brain results in bilirubin encephalopathy, which is also called _____.

C. Explain the underlying physiologic process that leads to hyperbilirubinemia in the newborn.

D. List the potential causes for pathologic jaundice or hyperbilirubinemia.

E. Identify the measures found to be effective in preventing hyperbilirubinemia.

F. Clinical manifestations of bilirubin encephalopathy or _____ typically appear between _____ after birth. During the first phase of the disorder, the newborn is _____ and _____, with a poor _____ and depressed or absent _____. These signs are followed by the appearance of a _____, _____, _____, and _____. Often _____ and _____ occur. These signs occur over a period of _____ hours. About _____ of the affected infants survive but many suffer from permanent neurologic sequelae.

2. Angela, who is Rh negative, had a spontaneous abortion at 13 weeks gestation, which resulted in what she said was just a heavier than usual menstrual period. Six months later she becomes pregnant again.

A. Describe the physiologic basis for Rh incompatibility and the occurrence of sensitization.

B. An indirect Coombs' test is positive. State the meaning of this finding.

C. Indicate if Angela is or is not a candidate for RhoGAM. Support your answer.

D. Describe RhoGAM (Rh immunoglobulin) and its use.

3. Baby girl Jennifer was born with spina bifida cystica and myelomeningocele. Describe the measures the nurse should use to manage Jennifer's care and help her parents cope with this congenital anomaly.

4. Baby girl Susan was born 2 hours ago. Her mother tested positive for HBsAg antibodies as a result of infection with hepatitis B virus (HBV).
   A. Describe the protocol that should be followed in providing care for Susan.

   B. Susan's mother asks the nurse if she can breastfeed her baby daughter. Discuss the nurse's response to this mother's question.

5. Baby boy Andrew is a full-term newborn who was just born by spontaneous vaginal delivery. Genital herpes recurred in his mother, and her membranes ruptured before the onset of labor.
   A. Identify the four modes of transmission for herpes simplex virus to the newborn. Indicate the mode most likely to have transmitted the infection to Andrew.

   B. List the clinical signs Andrew would exhibit as evidence of an active infection.

C. Describe the recommended nursing measures related to each of the following:
Care measures for Andrew and his parents

Vidarabine or acyclovir therapy

6. Baby girl Mary is 1 day old. Her mother's test for human immunodeficiency virus (HIV) is positive.
   A. Discuss Mary's potential for HIV infection and the possible modes of transmission.

   B. Mary's cord blood will most likely test _____ for the human immunodeficiency virus antibody. Diagnosis of HIV infection could be made when Mary is as young as _____ old if a combination of tests are used or as late as _____ old.
   C. Name the two opportunistic infections that, if contracted by Mary, would strongly suggest that she is infected with HIV.

   D. The average age for the onset of an opportunistic infection is _____ of age.

   E. Describe the care measures recommended for Mary.

   F. Mary's mother wishes to breastfeed Mary because she has read that it can prevent infection. Discuss the nurse's response to this mother's question.

7. Thomas, a 2-day-old breastfed infant, has developed oral candidiasis (thrush).
   A. Describe the signs most likely exhibited by Thomas that led to this diagnosis.

   B. Name the modes of transmission for this infection.

   C. Discuss the care management required by Thomas as a result of his fungal infection.

8. Jane, a newborn, has been diagnosed with fetal alcohol syndrome (FAS) as a result of moderate to sometimes heavy binge drinking by her mother throughout pregnancy.
   A. Describe the characteristics Jane most likely exhibited for the diagnosis of FAS to have been established.

   B. State three long-term effects Jane could experience as she gets older.

   C. Describe two nursing measures that could be effective in promoting Jane's growth and development.

9. Maternal substance abuse can be harmful to fetal and newborn health status, as well as growth and development.

    A. Describe the assessment findings associated with newborn withdrawal from each of the following substances:

    Heroin

    Methadone

    B. Identify the effects exhibited by newborns who have been exposed to cocaine while in utero.

    C. List the signs associated with neonatal abstinence syndrome.

    D. Describe the care management of mothers and of their infants who are affected by maternal substance abuse.

Answer Key

Chapter 1: Contemporary Maternity Nursing

Chapter Review Activities

1. C

2. H

3. D

4. F

5. A

6. G

7. B

8. E

9. Maternity nursing

10. Evidence based practice

11. Outcomes-oriented care, cost, length of stay, patient satisfaction

12. Managed care

13. Self care

14. Standards of care

15. Telemedicine

16. *Identify factors related to infant mortality:* Limited maternal education, young maternal age, unmarried, poverty, lack of prenatal care, poor nutrition, smoking, alcohol, and drug use, poor maternal health status

17. *Major changes in childbirth practices:* Nurse midwives, family-centered care, LDR/LDRPs, early discharge, neonatal security systems

18. *Barriers to prenatal care in US:* Inability to pay, lack of transportation, dependent child care, minority status, young maternal age, homeless

19. T

20. T

21. F

22. T

23. F

24. T

25. F

26. T

27. F

28. T

29. T

30. T

31. T

32. F

33. F

Critical Thinking Exercises

1. *Nursing director of inner city prenatal clinic:* See Trends in fertility and birth rate section, Box 1-1, and Table 1-1: answer should include:
   - biostatistics and contributing factors
   - factors associated with high-risk pregnancy (High-risk pregnancies escalate section)
   - impact of inadequate prenatal care (Access to care problems section)
   - importance of self care and ways to encourage participate in prenatal care (Trend toward consumer involvement and Self-care sections)

2. *High-technology care will not reduce rate of preterm birth and LBW infants:* See sections that cover the following topics to formulate answer:
   - factors associated with LBW and IMR
   - factors that escalate rate of high-risk pregnancy
   - high-tech care: what it can and cannot do

3. *Three proposed changes with rationale:* changes proposed should reflect efforts toward improving access to care, using research-based approaches and standards to guide care, and creating health-care services that address the factors associated with poor pregnancy outcomes.

4. *Self-care approaches:* use the information found in the Trends toward consumer involvement and Self-care section to formulate answer.

Chapter 2: The Family and Culture

Chapter Review Activities

1. B

2. E

3. D

4. C

5. F

6. A

7. Ethnocentrism

8. Acculturation

9. Assimilation

10. Subculture

11. Cultural relativism

12. Culture

13. Cultural context

14. Cultural competence

15. Family Functions: affective, socialization, reproductive, economic, health care

16. Family Dynamics: negotiation, boundaries, channels

17. Family Systems Theory

18. Family Developmental Theory

19. Family Stress Theory: internal, external

20. T

21. F

22. F

23. F

24. T

25. T

26. T

27. T

28. *List family functions and examples of each:* affective, socialization, reproductive, economic, health care

29. *Family theories:* see specific Family Theory sections for full description of each theory when formulating answer.

30. *Discuss how to consider products of culture when providing care:*
   - communication: consider language, need for a translator, dialect, style, and volume of speech, meaning of touch and gestures
   - space: include feelings of territoriality (varies), comfort zone must be established in terms of touch, proximity to others, handling of possessions, client must be in control of personal space to ensure a sense of autonomy and security
   - time: consider past, present, and future orientations and how this could effect meeting appointments, and health-care practices, beliefs, and goals
   - family roles: parent role, roles for grandparents, father's participation in pregnancy, labor, birth, and child care

31. *Identify factors that influence woman/family's adherence to cultural beliefs and practices:* individual subculture within the primary group, degree of acculturation, income level, amount of contact with older generations.

32. A

33. A

34. C

35. B

36. D

Crossword puzzle

Across: 2. Custom, 6. Socialization, 8. Family systems, 11. Culture, 12. Relativism, 13. Nuclear, 14. Future, 15. Extended, 17. Space, 19. Acculturation, 20. Health care
Down: 1. Subculture, 3. Family, 4. Economic, 5. Dynamics, 7. Assimilation, 8. Family stress, 9. Ethnocentrism, 10. Past oriented, 16. Developmental, 18. Channels

Critical Thinking Exercises

1. *Imagine you are a nurse working in a multicultural prenatal clinic:* Use Table 2-2 to formulate an answer related to Hispanic, African-American, and Asian women/families; consider the components of communication, space, time, roles; identify the degree to which each woman/family adheres to cultural beliefs and practices; do not stereotype

2. Pamela, a pregnant Native-American woman:
   A. *Questions to ask:* see questions listed in the Cultural Considerations section
   B. *Communication approach to use:* see Childbearing beliefs and practices subsection of Cultural Factors section; include concepts of communication patterns, space, time, and family roles when formulating answer
   C. *Identify Native American beliefs and practices:* see Table 2-2 to formulate answer; remember to determine her individual beliefs and practices—do not stereotype

3. Martinez family—recent birth of twin girls:
   A. *Identify family life stage:* family with young children; accepting new members into the system

B. *Developmental tasks of this stage:* See Table 2-1 for full list of the tasks this family must accomplish

C. *Describe cultural beliefs and practices:* Table 2-2 outlines parenting guidelines for several ethnic groups including those Hispanic families tend to follow

4. Refugee couple from Bosnia-prenatal care:
   - consider the process of working with a translator as outlined in Box 2-1; be sure to show respect for this couple by addressing the questions and comments to them and not to the translator
   - Box 2-1 outlines the preparation measures, interaction during the interview, and consultation with the translator after the interview
   - consult Chapter 3 for information regarding the stressors faced by refugees and the health-care needs they present
   - research Bosnia: cultural beliefs and practices and current political turmoil that led this couple to come to the United States

Chapter 3: Community and Home Care
Chapter Review Activities

1. F

2. T

3. F

4. T

5. T

6. F

7. T

8. T

9. T

10. F

11. F

12. T

13. T

14. F

15. F

16. F

17. T

18. people, place, interaction, or function

19. People, economics, recreation, physical environment, education, safety and transportation, politics and government, health and social services, communication

20. Census data, population size, age, sex, ethnic, socioeconomic, educational, employment, housing

21. aggregates

22. Primary prevention, immunizations, infant car seats

23. Secondary prevention, health screening

24. Tertiary prevention

25. Vulnerable populations, homeless, migrants, refugees, immigrants

26. *Indicators to assess community health and well-being:* to answer A and B see Box 3-1, which lists each category of indicators

27. *Identify five special population groups vulnerable to reproductive health risks:* pregnant adolescents, substance abusers, violence-prone families, mentally ill, persons with STDs or other communicable diseases, and those with malnutrition

28. *Cite the problems faced by migrant laborers/families:* See Migrants subsection; include in answer such problems as financial instability, child labor, poor housing and education, cultural barriers, limited access to services, hazardous work conditions, domestic violence, health problems such as diabetes, hypertension, malnutrition, tuberculosis, and substance abuse

29. *Three characteristics of refugees that increase their vulnerability:* see characteristics listed in the Refugees and immigrants subsection

30. *Identify factors that make home care a growth area:* these factors are fully listed in Current trends and historic perspectives subsection of Home Care along with the Perinatal continuum of care section

31. *Describe ways nurses can use the telephone to provide services:* see Telephonic nursing care subsection

32. *State advantages/disadvantages of perinatal home visits:*
advantages: natural setting, vulnerable newborn is protected, bedrest can be maintained, easier to observe and interact with the family, able to assess resources and safety, less expensive than hospital
disadvantages: increased time commitment for the nurse, more expensive than an office visit, limited availability of qualified nurses, nurse safety issues

33. *Identify home visit safety and infection control issues nurses must address:* see Safety issues for home care nurse and Infection control subsections of Plan of Care and Interventions for full discussion of safety and infection control

Critical Thinking Exercises

1. Home care nurse must become familiar with neighborhoods and their resources:
   A. *Windshield survey:* walking survey involving use of observations skills during a trip through a community
   B. *Use of findings:* see Table 3-1, which discusses each of the survey's components; describe how each of these components could reflect a community's strengths and problems; try using the survey to assess your community and the community in which your college is located.

2. Marie, a single parent of two children, homeless (see Homeless subsection):
   A. *Discuss types of health problems to which they are most vulnerable:* infections, anemia and other nutritionally related disorders, obesity, injury
   B. *Marie's vulnerability to becoming pregnant again:* victimization, economic survival, lack of access to health-care and birth-control measures, need for closeness and intimacy, doubt of fertility
   C. *Principles to guide nurse:* treat with respect and dignity, case management to coordinate care to meet multiple needs, flexible appointment times providing service when they come, make each interaction count, be purposeful, keep her empowered, help her to reconnect with her support system

3. Consuelo, pregnant wife of a migrant worker and mother of two (see Migrants subsection):
   • begin by confirming that she is pregnant
   • consider risks she faces including an increased rate of spontaneous abortion, inadequate prenatal care, and increased IMR as well as exposure to

teratogens; inadequate use of contraceptives, increased rate of STDs
including HIV, and poor nutrition are
also major concerns that need to be
addressed

4. *List questions for a postpartum follow-up
telephone call:* see Telephonic nursing care
subsection; include questions related to
how she is feeling and managing; the condition of her newborn and how it is eating,
eliminating, and sleeping; response of
other family members to the newborn; and
sources of happiness, stress, and
support/help

5. *Home visit to postpartum woman at 36
hours after birth:* See Box 3-2 and Care
management—the first home visit section
to answer each component of this exercise,
including the approach you would take to
prepare, your actions during the visit, how
you would end the visit, and the interventions you would follow after the visit,
including documentation of assessments,
actions, and responses.

6. *Angela, a pregnant woman with hyperemesis gravidarum:* see Health care along
the perinatal continuum of care: patient
selection and referral section for A and B
and Care management and interventions
subsection for C.
   A. *Criteria for discharge readiness:*
   Answer should include criteria related
   to Angela's health status and that of her
   fetus, availability of qualified home
   care professionals, family resources,
   and cost effectiveness of sending her
   home.
   B. *Information needed to institute high-
   tech care in the home:* medical diagnosis and prognosis, treatment required,
   medication history, drug dosing information, and type of infusion access
   device that will be used.

C. *Home environment criteria:* safe place
to store medications and infusion supplies; do a walk-through inspection to
determine temperature of the home,
general cleanliness, adequacy of area to
prepare and administer prescribed
treatment.

Chapter 4: Health Promotion and Prevention

Chapter Review Activities

1. Preconception care (see Preconception
   Counseling Section and Box 4-1 to formulate answer)
   A. *Describe preconception care:* helps
   couples to avoid unintended pregnancy; guides risk management so harmful
   behaviors can be changed to those that
   promote well being since the first
   trimester is critical for fetal development—women may not even know
   they are pregnant
   B. *List purposes:* identify and treat problems so they do not recur; minimize
   fetal malformation; behavior modifica-
   tion and risk reduction
   C. *Components:* Health promotion, Risk
   factor assessment, Interventions
   D. *Individuals who should participate:* all
   women of childbearing age; women
   who have had problems with a previous
   pregnancy; men who plan a pregnancy
   with their partner

2. *Identify reasons for seeking health care:*
   preconception care and counseling, pregnancy, well-woman care, fertility control,
   infertility treatment, menstrual problems,
   perimenopause

3. F

4. T

5. F

6. F

7. T

8. T

9. F

10. T

11. F

12. F

13. F

14. F

15. F

16. T

17. T

18. F

19. T

20. T

21. F

22. T

23. F

24. F

25. T

26. F

27. F

28. T

29. *Goals of prenatal care:* the major goals of prenatal care are listed in Box 4-2

30. *Components of well-woman care:* see Well-woman care section: include health assessment; age-appropriate screening; health promotion; support from health-care provider; holistic approach that considers culture, religion, age, personal differences

31. *Identify changes associated with the climacteric:* see Perimenopause section and Box 4-4 for full description of changes experienced by women

32. *Barriers to seeking health care:* see Barriers to seeking health care section; address financial, cultural, and gender issues

33. *Impact of illicit drugs on the maternal-fetal unit:* see Illicit drug subsection of Health behaviors section; consider effects of cocaine, heroin, marijuana

34. Anorexia nervosa, strict/severe diets, vigorous extreme exercise, depression

35. Bulimia nervosa, self induced vomiting, laxatives, diuretics, strict diets, fasting, vigorous exercise

36. Wife battering, spouse abuse, domestic, family violence, physical, sexual, psychologic, economic, pregnancy

37. repeated, increasing tension, battery, calm and remorse, honeymoon

38. 18, 3 years, disrobing, nudity, masturbation, fondling, digital penetration, anal, oral, vaginal

39. Incest, 18, sexual assault

40. Rape, penile penetration, sex organ, labia, acquaintance, marital, gang, stranger, psychic, sexual assault, touch, kisses, hugs, petting, intercourse, sexual

41. *List consequences of STDs:* infertility, ectopic pregnancy, neonatal morbidity and mortality, genital cancer, AIDS, death

42. *Identify risks for gynecologic cancers:* see Risks for gynecologic cancers subsection of Gynecologic conditions affecting pregnancy section; several risk factors for cervical, endometrial, and ovarian cancers are identified

43. *Compare characteristics of women in abusive and nonviolent relationships:*
    abusive: nurturing, compassionate, sympathetic, yielding, more willing to tolerate control, social isolation, low self-esteem
    nonviolent: assertive, independent, willing to take a stand

44. *List long-term effects experienced by incest survivors:* see Sexual abuse subsection for lists of physical symptoms/effects and psychosocial symptoms/effects

Crossword puzzle

Across: 1. Endometrial; 3. Climacteric; 4. Osteoporosis; 6. Spermicide; 8. Contraception; 9. Abortion; 11. IUD; 13. Mammogram; 14. Puberty; 15. Prostaglandins; 16. Menstruation; 17. Condom; 18. Metrorrhagia; 20. Sterilization; 21. Leiomyoma; 22. Menarche; 23. Menorrhagia

Down: 1. Endometriosis; 2. Diaphragm; 5. Preconception; 7. Infertility; 10. Papanicolaou; 12. Dysmenorrhea; 16. Menopause; 19. Ovarian

Critical Thinking Exercises

1. *Process of preconception counseling:*
   • explain importance of preparing for pregnancy and how critical it is to be in good health and follow good health habits in the first trimester even before you know you are pregnant, implement the components of preconception care (Box 4-1)
   • include George in counseling and care

2. *Describe approach for well-woman care with woman who is anxious and embarrassed:*
   • support and reassurance from the first contact so she will feel comfortable coming for care in the future; serious concerns may surface
   • coordinate her care—ensure all appropriate services are provided, assessment completed, and health guidance given; consider that this may be her only contact with the health-care system
   • sensitive interviewing and careful, respectful examination since she may be embarrassed by her signs and symptoms

3. *Teenage pregnant woman seeking prenatal care:* see Age—Teenage pregnancy section
   A. *Risk related to adolescent pregnancy:* may be noncompliant with nutrition and prenatal care; additional stress related to being impulsive, self-centered, peer oriented; risk for preterm labor and birth, IUGR, PIH; single status, long-term effects of disrupted education, infant-related risks occur as well
   B. *Approach of nurse who provides prenatal care:* full holistic assessment and approach that includes Suzanne's family and boyfriend; use developmental principles related to adolescence to guide care; involve her support system, provide incentives for participation in prenatal care and health-care regimen, refer to community services as needed

4. *Pregnant woman who smokes:*
   • discuss impact of smoking on pregnancy using statistics, illustrations, research, and case studies to convince her of the harmful effects of her habit on her, her pregnancy, and her baby before and after it is born; see Smoking subsection of Health behaviors section and Box 4-5

- help her to change her behavior by referring her to smoking cessation programs; use motivation of pregnancy to at least limit smoking if she cannot stop completely. See Substance use subsection of Anticipatory guidance for health promotion and prevention section

5. *Health promotion and prevention class for a group of young adult women:*
   A. *Content outline:* see individual subsections for nutrition, exercise, and health-risk prevention found in Anticipatory guidance for health promotion and prevention section; consider forming support groups for women who wish to change behaviors using the concept of a "buddy system" to facilitate positive, long-lasting change.
   B. *Meaning of safer sex:* discuss meaning of risking behavior, consequences of infections and how to prevent them; see Box 4-8.
   C. *Measures to protect self from violence and injury:* discuss protective and legal services including resources and hotlines (Box 4-9); facilitate access, promote assertiveness, refer to self-defense courses, support and self-help groups, educate to develop independence; see Health protection section.

6. *Woman experiencing stress:*
   A. *Identify effects of stress:* see Box 4-6 for list of physical and emotional effects of stress.
   B. *Stress management techniques:*
      - identify sources of stress and measures that can be used to reduce the stress from these sources
      - discuss stress relievers, time management skills, relaxation exercises, use of biofeedback and guided imagery; role play
      - see Stress management subsection in Anticipatory guidance for health promotion and prevention section

Chapter 5: Health Assessment

Chapter Review Activities

1. mons pubis

2. labia majora

3. labia minora

4. prepuce

5. frenulum

6. fourchette

7. clitoris

8. vestibule

9. perineum

10. vagina, rugae

11. fornices

12. squamocolumnar junction

13. fundus

14. endometrium

15. myometrium

16. uterine (fallopian) tubes

17. ovaries, ovulation, estrogen, progesterone, androgen

18. *Label illustrations:*
    A. *External female genitalia* (Fig. 5-1): A, mons pubis, B, prepuce of clitoris, C, frenulum of clitoris, D, labia minora, E, Skene's duct opening, F, Bartholin's duct opening, G, vestibule, H, fourchette, I, posterior commissure, J, perineum, K, anus, L, fossa navicularis, M, hymen, N, vaginal orifice, O, labia

majora, P, vestibule, Q, urethra, R, glans of clitoris, S, anterior commissure

B. *Perineal body:* A, posterior fornix, B, buttocks, C, rectum, D, anus, E, perineal body, F, vagina, G, urethra, H, symphysis pubis, I, bladder, J, uterus, K, cul de sac of Douglas

C. *Cross section of uterus, adnexa, and upper vagina:* A, fundus, B, body (corpus) of uterus, C, endometrium, D, myometrium, E, internal os of the cervix, F, external os of the cervix, G, vagina, H, endocervical canal, I, fornix of vagina, J, cardinal ligament, K, uterine blood vessels, L, broad ligament, M, ovary, N, fimbriae, O, infundibulum of uterine tube, P, ampulla, Q, ovarian ligament, R, isthmus of uterine tube, S, interstitial portion of uterine tube

D. *Female breast (sagittal section):* A, clavicle, B, intercostal muscle, C, pectoralis major, D, alveolus, E, ductule, F, duct, G, lactiferous duct, H, lactiferous sinus, I, nipple pore, J, suspensory ligament of Cooper, K, sixth rib, L, second rib. *Female breast (anterior dissection):* A, acini cluster, B, lactiferous (milk) ducts, C, lactiferous sinus ampulla, D, nipple pore, E, areola, F, Montgomery's tubercle

E. *Female pelvis:* A, seventh lumbar vertebra, B, iliac crest, C, sacral promontory, D, sacrum, E, acetabulum, F, obturator foramen, G, subpubic arch under symphysis pubis, H, ischium, I, pubis, J, ilium, K, sacroiliac joint

19. A. *Label diagram of menstrual cycle:* (Fig. 5-7) A, gonadotrophin releasing hormone, B, FSH, C, LH, D, follicular phase, E, luteal phase, F, graafian follicle, G, ovum, H, corpus luteum, I, estrogen, J, progesterone, K, menstruation, L, proliferative phase, M, secretory phase, N, ischemic phase,

O, hypothalamic-pituitary cycle, P, ovarian cycle, Q, endometrial cycle

B. *Describe events in each cycle composing the menstrual cycle:* see Hypothalamic-pituitary cycle, Ovarian cycle, and Endometrial cycle subsections of Menstruation section for full description of the events and changes characteristic of each cycle.

C. *Identify cyclical changes:*
- basal body temperature: falls just prior to ovulation then rises after ovulation as a result of increasing level of progesterone.
- preovulatory and postovulatory mucous is viscous to prevent sperm penetration but ovulatory mucous is thin, clear, stretchy, and alkaline to support sperm viability and facilitate penetration.

20. F

21. F

22. T

23. T

24. F

25. F

26. F

27. T

28. F

29. F

30. T

31. T

32. *State how culture, age, physical and emotional disorders, abuse can influence health assessment of women:* see Cultural and communication variables, Age-related,

considerations, Women with special needs, and Abused women subsections in the Health assessment section.

33. *Instructions for a Pap smear:* see Procedure Box—Papanicolaou smear for preparation guidelines related to douching, use of vaginal preparations, intercourse, and menstruation.

34. *Describe function of various hormones:* see the following subsections in the Menstruation section for full information on each hormone: hypothalamic-pituitary cycle (Gn-RH, FSH, LH), ovarian cycle (estrogen and progesterone) and prostaglandins.

35. *Complete table related to the sexual response cycle:* see Table 5-2.

36. B

37. D

38. A

39. H

40. F

41. C

42. I

43. E

44. G

45. *Description of pelvic examination:* each component of the examination is fully described in a separate subsection of the Pelvic examination section.

46. *Guidelines for performing a Pap smear:* guidelines for each component of the procedures are outlined in the Procedure Box—Papanicolaou Smear.

Critical Thinking Exercises

1. Answering questions and concerns of women expressed to the nurse who is providing health care:
   A. *Hymen:* hymen can be perforated with strenuous exercise, insertion of tampons, masturbation, gynecologic examination as well as during vaginal intercourse.
   B. *Signs indicative of ovulation:* mid-cycle bleeding and pain (Mittelschmerz), breast swelling and tenderness, elevated basal body temperature, cervical mucous changes (spinnbarkeit), and other changes in behavior and emotions individual to each woman (premenstrual signs).
   C. *Breast characteristics across the life span:* see Table 5-1, which outlines characteristics of the breasts of adolescent, adult, and postmenopausal women.
   D. *Douching:* vaginal secretions are usually slightly acidic and protect the vagina from infection; a douche may alter this acidity and injure the mucosa, thereby increasing the risk for infection; regular front to back washing with soap and water is all that is necessary to be clean.

2. *Conducting a health history interview of a female patient:*
   A. *Writing questions to use:* use Health history outline in the Health assessment section as a guide for question areas; questions should be open-ended, clear, concise, and progress from the general to the specific.
   B. *Therapeutic communication techniques with examples:* use facilitation, reflection, clarification, empathetic responses, confrontation, interpretation.

3. *Teaching self-examination techniques:* since each technique involves cognitive,

psychomotor, and affective learning, a variety of methodologies must be used including: discussion of technique—when and how often to do, why it should be done, what is normal and abnormal, who to call if changes are noted, what will happen to determine basis of the change, and feelings regarding performance—literature, demonstration and redemonstration, videos and illustration, breast models, guest speakers of women who have used the techniques successfully for early detection and prompt treatment.

   A. *Breast Self-Examination:* see Home Care Box for full explanation of the technique.

   B. *Vulvar (genital) Self-Examination:* see External palpation subsection of the Pelvic examination section for a full explanation of the technique.

4. *Culturally sensitive approach to women's health care:*
   - approach woman in a respectful and calm manner
   - consider modifications in the examination to maintain her modesty
   - incorporate communication variations such as conversational style, pacing, space, eye contact, touch, time orientation
   - take time to learn about the woman's cultural beliefs and practices regarding well-woman care

5. *Screening for abuse when providing well woman care:*
   - A. *Adjusting the environment:* provide for comfort and privacy, assess the woman alone without her partner or adult children present.
   - B. *Abuse indicators:* Box 5-1 lists indications of abuse and areas of the body most commonly injured, including head, neck, chest, abdomen, breasts, and upper extremities; note location and patterns of bruises and burns and specific somatic complaints.

   C. *Questions to ask:* Figure 5-10 lists four questions that **ALL** women should be asked.

   D. *Approach if abuse is confirmed:*
   - acknowledge the abuse and affirm that it is unacceptable and common; tell her you are concerned and that she does not deserve it.
   - communicate that it can reoccur; discuss the cycle of violence and that help is available; empower the woman to use the help that is available to her and her children.
   - help her to formulate an escape plan.

6. *Assisting with a pelvic examination:* see Procedure Box—Assisting with Pelvic Examination and Pelvic examination section of the text to formulate the answer.
   - woman should be taught about what is going to occur as part of the examination, assisted to change clothes and to get into the position required for the examination; inform and support woman during the examination and provide privacy; assist with cleansing, getting into an upright position, and dressing after the examination; discuss any questions and concerns the woman might have relate to the examination.
   - assist with preparing and supporting the patient, preparing equipment, and taking care of specimens.

Chapter 6: Common Health Problems

Chapter Review Activities

1. Amenorrhea, pregnancy, anorexia nervosa

2. Dysmenorrhea, onset of menstruation, primary dysmenorrhea, 6 to 12 months, ovulation, estrogen, progesterone, secondary dysmenorrhea, a few days after menses begins

3. Premenstrual syndrome, symptoms occur in the luteal phase and resolve within a few days of the onset of menstruation, symptom-free period occurs in the follicular phase, symptoms are recurrent

4. Endometriosis, proliferative, secretory, menstruation, inflammatory, fibrosis, adhesions, dysmenorrhea, diarrhea, pain with defecation, constipation, infertility

5. Oligomenorrhea, hypomenorrhea, oral contraceptive pill (OCP)

6. Metrorrhagia, intermenstrual bleeding, OCPs, Norplant, IUDs

7. Menorrhagia, hypermenorrhea, hormonal disturbances, systemic diseases, benign and malignant neoplasms, infection, contraception, non steroidal anti-inflammatory drugs (NSAIDs)

8. Dysfunctional uterine bleeding (DUB), anovulation, LH, progesterone, corpus luteum, extremes of a woman's reproductive years, menarche, menopause, hormonal, estrogen, progesterone

9. T

10. F

11. T

12. T

13. F

14. F

15. F

16. T

17. T

18. F

19. T

20. F

21. F

22. T

23. T

24. F

25. T

26. F

27. F

28. F

29. T

30. F

31. T

32. *Hypogonadotropic amenorrhea:* see appropriate subsection of Menstrual problems section.
A. *Risk factors:* stress, inappropriate body fat-to-lean ratio, athletic training, eating disorders
B. *Nurse's role:* counseling and education regarding stress reduction, appropriate nutrition, balanced exercise programs, sensible weight loss; discuss substance abuse issues; educate regarding prescribed medications including OCPs and calcium

33. *List signs and symptoms associated with PMS:* consider major categories when formulating answer: fluid retention, behavioral and emotional changes, premenstrual cravings, discomforts; see PMS subsection of Menstrual problems section.

34. *Categorize sexual behaviors according to infection safety or risk:* see Table 6-2 to answer this question.

35. *List the most common STDs in women:* chlamydia, human papillomavirus, gonorrhea, herpes simplex II, syphilis, HIV.

36. *Complete table related to STDs and vaginal infections:* see Infection section for specific subsection for each infection listed on the table.

37. uterine tubes, uterus, ovaries, peritoneal

38. Chlamydia, one half, vagina, endocervix, upper genital tract, end of or just after menses following reception of the infectious agent, abortion, pelvic surgery, childbirth

39. ectopic pregnancy, infertility, chronic pelvic pain, dyspareunia, pyosalpinx, tubo-ovarian abscess, pelvic adhesions

40. pain, fever, chills, nausea and vomiting, increased vaginal discharge, symptoms of UTI, irregular bleeding

41. prevention, education to avoid STDs, preventing lower genital tract infections from ascending to the upper genital tract

42. *Risk factors for hepatitis B:* ethnic background, place of employment and job there, types of contacts with other persons such as family, friends, sexual partner.

43. *Heterosexual transmission of HIV to women:* see HIV infection section.
    A. *Mode of transmission:* exchange of body fluids
    B. *Signs and symptoms during seroconversion:* viremic, influenza-type responses such as fever, headache, night sweats, malaise, lymphadenopathy, myalgia, nausea, diarrhea, weight loss, sore throat, rash
    C. *Risk behaviors:* IV drug use, high-risk sexual partner, multiple sexual partners, history of multiple STDs
    D. *Management:* education, expert multidisciplinary care with a holistic focus,

referrals (psychologic, legal, financial), measures to prevent infection and maintain resistance, prophylactic medication; see Plan of care and interventions subsection

44. *State two precautions for Standard Precautions and Precautions for Invasive Procedures:* see Box 6-3, which describes several precautions for each category.

45. *Risk factors for breast cancer:* see Box 6-4 for a full list.

Critical Thinking Exercises

1. *Woman experiencing dysmenorrhea* (see Dysmenorrhea—primary subsection of Menstrual problems section)
   A. *Nursing diagnosis:* consider the areas of pain and altered role performance as the focus for nursing management of this woman's primary dysmenorrhea
   B. *Self-care measures:* discuss basis of problem and that it usually diminishes with age; suggest nonpharmacologic measures such as exercise, relaxation techniques, good nutrition, heating pad; pharmacologic measures such as NSAIDs and oral contraceptives may be ordered

2. *Woman with PMS—nursing approach:* obtain a detailed history and encourage the woman to keep a diary of physical and emotional manifestations (what occurs, when, circumstances) from one cycle to another; try to individualize a plan based on her experiences; discuss nutrition, exercise, and lifestyle/career measures; refer as appropriate to counseling and support groups.

3. *Woman with endometriosis* (see Endometriosis section).
   A. *Clinical manifestations:* dysmenorrhea, pelvic pain and heaviness, thigh pain, GI symptoms, dyspareunia, metrorrhagia/menorrhagia

B. *Pathophysiology of the disorder:* growth of endometrial tissue outside the uterus mainly in the pelvis—implants respond to cyclical changes in hormones—bleed leading to inflammatory response and formation of scar tissue/adhesions and fibrosis

C. *Pharmacologic management:* each pharmacologic approach is discussed in the Management subsection; oral contraceptives (create a pseudopregnancy and shrink implants), Gn-RH antagonists and androgenic synthetic steroids create a pseudomenopause

D. *Support measures:* education, discuss treatment options both pharmacologic and nonpharmacologic, refer to support groups and counseling as needed, work with the couple together and separately, review options for pregnancy since infertility can be an outcome

4. *Woman with pelvic inflammatory disease (PID):* see Pelvic Inflammatory disease section.

A. *Nursing management plan:*
- position/activity: bedrest in the semi-Fowlers position to keep pelvis in the dependent position; elevate legs slightly to prevent pulling on pelvis, which would increase discomfort
- comfort measures: analgesics, backrub, hygiene, relaxation techniques, diversional activities
- support measures: provide time for woman to discuss feelings, include partner in care as appropriate; help woman to deal with effects of the PID and the potential long-term effects; use a nonjudgmental, empathetic approach
- health education: how to comply with treatment regimen, including taking medications effectively, refraining from intercourse until fully healed, use of contraceptives, and safer sex measures

B. *Self-care during recovery phase:* see Home Care Box—STDs

5. *Measures to prevent transmission of hepatitis B virus:* immunoprophylaxis for household members and sexual contacts, maintain high level of personal hygiene, careful disposal of items contaminated with blood or body fluids including saliva, safer sex measures.

6. *Woman concerned regarding possible exposure to HIV.*
A. *Testing procedure:* see HIV testing and counseling subsection for full description of testing protocol, counseling required, and legal implications; nurse should witness an informed consent, tell the woman how long it will take for results to be available, consider ethical issues of confidentiality and privacy, and use a nonjudgmental, empathetic approach

B. *Counseling protocol:* counseling should occur before and after testing and be done by the same person; counseling should take place in a private area with no interruptions

7. *Woman with a lump in her left breast* (see Cancer of breast section).
A. *Diagnostic protocol:* clinical examination of the breast by health-care provider, mammography, needle aspiration/localization biopsy, laboratory testing (CBC, liver enzymes, serum Ca, alkaline phosphatase)

B. *Preoperative care measures:* answer should emphasize education and support including a visit from a woman who had the same procedure; implement typical preoperative physical care measures.
Immediate postoperative care measures: answer should emphasize establishing physiologic stability, taking care not to take BP, perform a venipuncture,

or give parenteral medications in the affected arm; care for dressing and drains, being alert for signs of hemorrhage (check drainage container and area under the patient for excessive bleeding)

C. *Self-care instructions for home:* see Home Care Box—Patient Instructions for Self-Care after a Mastectomy for identification of areas for health teaching to prepare woman to care for herself at home

D. *Support measures:*
- help woman and her partner deal with her change in appearance and self-concept; encourage open communication with nurse and each other; meet with woman and partner together and separately
- refer to community resources including Reach For Recovery
- discuss follow-up treatments that may be required such as chemotherapy and radiation
- discuss reconstructive surgery and use of prosthesis as is appropriate for this woman

Chapter 7: Contraception, Infertility, and Abortion

Chapter Review Activities

1. T
2. F
3. F
4. T
5. T
6. F
7. F
8. T
9. T
10. T
11. F
12. F
13. T
14. F
15. T
16. F
17. T
18. T
19. F

20. *Characteristics of ideal contraceptive:* safe, easily available, economical, acceptable, simple to use, promptly reversible

21. *Factors influencing effectiveness of contraceptive method:* see full list in Box 7-1.

22. *Meaning of BRAIDED:* benefits, risks, alternatives, inquires, decisions, explanations, documentation

23. A. exact time of ovulation cannot be predicted accurately, exercise restraint for several days, irregular menstrual periods
    B. 5, 22
    C. drop, 0.05°, progesterone, rise, 0.2° to 0.4°, 2 to 4 days, thermal shift, day of the drop in BBT, 3 days
    D. cervical mucus, cervical mucus, amount, consistency
    E. BBT, cervical mucus, increased libido, mid-cycle spotting, mittelschmerz, pelvic fullness, tenderness, vulvar fullness
    F. LH, 12 to 24

24. *Label as "C" correct or "I" incorrect*
    A. C
    B. C
    C. C
    D. I
    E. C
    F. I
    G. I

25. *Label as "C" correct or "I" incorrect*
    A. C
    B. I
    C. C
    D. C
    E. C
    F. I
    G. I
    H. I

26. *Cite four factors for seeking an abortion:* preserve life and health of the woman, genetic disorder of fetus, rape/incest, pregnant woman's request

27. T

28. T

29. F

30. T

31. F

32. T

33. T

34. T

35. *Couple makes first visit to fertility clinic* (see Infertility section and subsections)
    A. *Identify/describe components for normal fertility:* normal male and female reproductive tract, hormonal support for gametogenesis, timing of intercourse, adequate sperm and ova, patent tubal system for passage of sperm and ova

    B. *Support statement that assessment for infertility must involve both partners:* see Box 7-6, which outlines findings favorable for fertility indicating male and female factors; cite statistics revealing that a female factor causes 40 to 55%, a male factor causes 30 to 40%, a couple factor 10%, and unexplained 10%.

36. *Pharmacologic measures to treat infertility:* see Medical treatment subsection of Plan of care and interventions—infertility section for a full discussion of each of the medication listed.

37. *Infertility:* never been pregnant, never impregnated a woman, been pregnant at least once but has not been able to conceive again or sustain a pregnancy.
    Causes for female and male infertility: see specific subsections in Infertility section for full listing

38. E

39. C

40. B

41. D

42. A

43. F

44. *Alternative birth technologies:*
    A. *Definitions of each type:* see Table 7-4.
    B. *Ethical issues:* see Box 7-9, which identifies ethical issues and ethical questions related to the use of alternative birth technologies.

Critical Thinking Exercises

1. *Discuss approach to use when woman seeks information about birth control:*
   - assess her level of knowledge regarding how her body works and different methods; determine her and/or her

partner's preferences for and objections to specific measures; fully discuss methods preferred or not known to the woman and/or her partner

- sexual practices: beliefs and preferences, number of partners, frequency of coitus
- level of contraceptive involvement: comfort with touching genitalia, myths and misconceptions, religious and cultural factors
- health status as determined during a thorough health history interview, physical examination, and laboratory testing as appropriate

2. *Woman choosing to use combination estrogen-progestin oral contraceptive:*
   A. *Mode of action:* suppression of hypothalamus and anterior pituitary, altered maturation of the endometrium, and thickened cervical mucus
   B. *Advantages of use:* easy to take at same time of day, not directly related to sexual act, improved sexual response, regular predicable menses with decrease blood loss, decrease dysmenorrhea and PMS, protection from endometrial and possibly ovarian cancer
   C. *Absolute contraindications:* history of thrombophlebitis, cerebrovascular or coronary artery disease, breast cancer, estrogen dependent tumor, pregnancy, impaired liver function/tumor, undiagnosed vaginal bleeding, smokers >35 years. *Relative contraindications:* migraines, hypertension, elective surgery, epilepsy, sickle cell disease, diabetes, gallbladder disease
   D. *Cite side effects in terms of estrogen excess/deficiency and progestin excess/deficiency:* side effects are fully discussed in the Disadvantages and side effects subsection of Hormonal methods section
   E. *Signs and symptoms requiring woman to stop taking OCP and notify her health care provider:* see Signs of

Potential Complications box—oral contraceptives for full explanation of ACHES
   F. *Specify patient instructions:*
   - follow specific directions on package insert in terms of taking the pill and what to do if one or more are missed
   - use own pills not someone else's since OCPs vary
   - discuss side effects and complications
   - check effect of other medications being taken on the effectiveness of the OCP
   - importance of using STD protection and alternative method for the first cycle on the OCP

3. *Woman using a cervical cap:* use proper size and fit, when to insert and length of time it can and should stay in place, how to insert and to check placement, use of spermicide, do not use during menses.

4. *Instructions following insertion of IUD:* see Signs of Complications box—IUD which uses the acronym PAINS to identify signs of problems; teach woman how and when to check the string (after menses, at ovulation, and before coitus); inform woman when the IUD needs to be replaced.

5. *Couple contemplating sterilization:* see Sterilization section.
   A. *Decision-making approach:* nurse acts as a facilitator to help couple explore the pros and cons of sterilization itself and the methods available; nurse also provides information about each method.
   B. *Preoperative and postoperative care measures and instructions:*
   - preoperative period: holistic health assessment in terms of history, physical examination, and laboratory tests; discuss preparatory instructions, witness an informed consent

- postoperative period: prevention and early detection of bleeding and infection; self-care measures in terms of hygiene, comfort, reduction of swelling with ice packs, scrotal support, moderate activity restriction for a couple of days
- caution that sterility is not immediate: an alternative method must be used until sperm count is zero for two consecutive semen analyses; STD protection must be considered as appropriate

6. *Couple using symptothermal method of contraception:*
   A. *List components:* BBT, cervical mucus, secondary cycle phase related symptoms
   B. *Measuring BBT:* see Teaching Guidelines box—BBT and Fig. 7-1; *Evaluating cervical mucus characteristics:* see Teaching Guidelines box—cervical mucus characteristics
   C. *Effectiveness:* when abstinence is practiced during the fertile period the effectiveness ranges between 73% to 97%.

7. *Couple undergoing testing for infertility:*
   A. *Assessment of the woman and man:* see Boxes 7-5 and 7-7 for full explanation of the components of the assessment process for infertility
   B. *Procedure for semen analysis:* see Semen analysis subsection of Assessment of male infertility section; emphasize need to abstain for 2 to 5 days before the collection, not to use a spermicide, to bring the specimen to the laboratory within 2 hours of collection making sure to use a clean container, and not to expose the specimen to excessive heat or cold.
   C. *Semen characteristics:* see Box 7-8 for full list of expected characteristics in terms of liquification, volume, pH, density, morphology

   D. *Postcoital test instructions:* see Postcoital test subsection of Assessment of the couple section; instructions should include purpose of the test, when to have intercourse, what to do afterwards, when to come for examination; caution that vagina must be free of infection and couple should abstain for 2 to 4 days before the test.
   E. *Nursing support measures:* see Psychosocial subsection of Plan of care and interventions—infertility section; help couple to express feelings and to openly discuss sexuality issues; help the couple with the decision-making process; facilitate the grieving process when they determine that biologic children are not in their future; refer to support groups, adoption agencies as appropriate.

8. *Woman scheduled for diagnostic laparoscopy:* see Laparoscopy subsection of Diagnostic tests section.
   A. *Timing:* early in the menstrual cycle to avoid disturbing a fertilized ovum
   B. *Preoperative care measures:* NPO for 8 hours, void before the procedure, bowel preparation may be required
   C. *Purpose of the procedure:* diagnostic (visualize structures to determine if abnormalities are present) and therapeutic (surgery can be performed to relieve blockages, release adhesions, remove endometrial implants, etc.) purposes; small incisions will be made into the abdomen to allow passage of laparoscope; carbon dioxide will be inserted to allow visualization of pelvic structures.
   D. *Postoperative measures:* answer should discuss assessment of vital signs, LOC, incision sites, signs of bleeding, infection, pain, prevention of aspiration, administration of IV fluids, relief of discomfort, assist with elimination; discharge usually occurs within 4 to 6 hours; discharge instructions should

include expectations regarding referred shoulder pain for up to 12 hours related to the use of carbon dioxide, use of mild analgesic for pain, type of activity restriction, signs of infection and bleeding and who to call if such signs appear.

9. *Woman contemplating elective abortion:* see Care Management-Abortion section
   A. *Describe approach:* use therapeutic communication techniques to establish trusting relationship; discuss alternatives available to her and the consequences of each in terms of the woman's own values and beliefs; the nurse facilitates the decision-making process and the patient makes the decision; make appropriate referral to help her with the decision.
   B. *Purpose of laminaria and procedure for vacuum aspiration:* see Vacuum aspiration subsection of First Trimester Abortion; laminaria is used to dilate the cervix (2 to 24 hours) then procedure is performed (5 minutes).
   C. *Three nursing diagnoses:* consider decisional conflict and fear, then anticipatory grieving, risk for infection, and pain.
   D. *Nursing measures for care and support:* assess physical condition checking for bleeding and ability to void, keep her informed, provide support and comfort measures.
   E. *Discharge instructions:* hygiene measures to prevent infection: shower, avoid use of tampons and douches; identify signs and symptoms of complications (bleeding, infection), discuss activity restrictions, resumption of sexual relations, use of birth control and safer sex measures; arrange for follow-up appointment and stress its importance.

Chapter 8: Conception and Fetal Development
Chapter Review Activities

1. ovum, ovarian follicle, cilia, tube, 24

2. sperm, 4 to 6, 2 to 3, capacitation, enzymes, ampulla, impenetrable, zona reaction

3. nuclei, diploid, zygote, 3, morula, blastocyst, implanted, 6 to 10, decidua, chorionic villi, trophoblast, basalis

4. *Functions of yolk sac, amniotic fluid and membranes, umbilical cord, placenta:* see individual subsections for each structure in the Development of the Embryo section.

5. *Fetal circulation-shunts:* see Fetal circulatory system subsection in the Fetal maturation section; Fig. 8-9; discuss ductus venosus (liver bypass), ductus arteriosus (lung bypass), foramen ovale (between the atria; lung bypass).

6. T

7. F

8. T

9. T

10. F

11. F

12. T

13. F

14. F

15. T

16. F

17. T

18. T

19. F

20. F

21. T

22. F

23. *Genetic counseling:* see Genetic counseling section for full discussion of each section of this question
    A. *Purpose:*
       - advise couple before conception of the probability of conception of an infant with a genetic disorder
       - advise couple after conception and fetal screening of whether the fetus has a genetic disorder
       - inform couple of options available
    B. *Estimation of risk:* use of Mendelian principles for disorders caused by a specific factor that segregate during cell division (unifactorial inheritance); estimation of risk for multifactorial inheritance is much less accurate. *Interpretation of risk:* explanation of risk to the couple without giving advice; couple makes decision, not the health-care provider.
    C. *Nurse's role in genetic counseling:* clarify information and provide follow-up care that includes providing emotional support and referring the couple to agencies and support groups related to their specific genetic disorder.

24. *Complete table related to primary germ layers:* see Primary germ layers subsection of the embryo and fetus section for identification of tissues and organs that develop from each layer.

25. *Factors that determine risk for inheritable disorder:* health status of family members, abnormal reproductive outcomes, history of maternal disorders, drug exposures, and illnesses, advanced maternal and paternal age, and ethnic origin

26. *Explain each type of inheritance and give example:*
    - Unifactorial inheritance: inheritable characteristic is controlled by a single gene; recessive or dominant
    - Multifactorial inheritance: congenital disorder resulting from a combination of genetic and environmental factors
    - X-linked inheritance: transmission of abnormal genes on the X-chromosome; both males and females can be affected but tends to be less severe in females since they also have a normal gene on their second X-chromosome

Critical Thinking Exercises

1. Questions from prenatal clients to nurse midwives:
    A. *Progress of fetal development at 2 months, 5 months, and 7 months:* See Table 8-1 to formulate answer; use of illustrations and life-size models would facilitate learning.
    B. *Survival after 35 weeks gestation:* Discuss how the respiratory system develops including the critical factor of surfactant production; describe how surfactant helps the newborn to breathe.
    C. *Quickening:* Explain that this is the woman's perception of fetal movement that occurs at about 16 to 20 weeks gestation; use Box 8-2 to describe how the fetus moves; it will not hurt but can interfere with her rest toward the end of her pregnancy; fetus will develop its own sleep-wake cycles.
    D. *Fetal sensory perception:* Discuss sensory capability of the fetus using Sensory awareness subsection of the Fetal maturation section; fetus can hear sounds such as parents' voices and can respond to light touch.

E. *Sex determination:* Discuss function of the X and Y chromosome; inform her that sex of fetus becomes recognizable around 12 weeks gestation.

F. *Multiple gestation—twins:* Discuss monozygotic (identical) and dizygotic (fraternal) twinning and how each occurs; emphasize that fraternal-type twinning tends to occur in families.

2. *Couple facing a genetic disorder:*

A. *Process to determine genetic risk:* Tay Sachs is an autosomal-recessive disorder that follows a unifactorial inheritance pattern; Mr. Goldberg needs to be tested since he must also be a carrier to produce a child with the disorder; emphasize nurse's role in terms of emotional support, facilitation of the decision making process, and interpretation of diagnostic test results and how they can influence future childbearing decisions.

B. *Inheritance possibility when both parents carry a recessive gene:* Since both parents are carriers of a recessive gene, there is a one in four chance the child will be normal, two in four chance the child will be a carrier because they are, and one in four chance the child will have the disorder; this inheritance pattern is the same for every pregnancy; there is no reduction or increase in risk from one pregnancy to another.

C. *Decision-making process for this couple:* Discuss nature of this disorder, extent of risk and consequences if the child inherits the disorder, options available related to pregnancy, use of amniocentesis to determine if child is affected, continuing with the pregnancy or having an abortion, using reproductive technology, adopting, or remaining childless.

Crossword puzzle

Across: 1. HCG; 3. umbilical cord; 9. implantation; 11. chromosome; 12. amniotic; 13. surfactant; 15. dizygotic; 17. mutation; 18. genome; 19. ductus arteriosus; 21. gene; 23. meiosis; 24. chorionic villi; 26. monozygotic; 27. karyotype; 28. teratogen

Down: 2. cephalocaudal; 4. blastocyst; 5. conception; 6. viability; 7. gamete; 8. zygote; 10. morula; 14. fetus; 15. decidua basalis; 16. foramen ovale; 20. fertilization; 22. placenta; 25. embryo

Chapter 9: Anatomy and Physiology of Pregnancy
Chapter Review Activities

1. gravidity

2. parity

3. gravida

4. nulligravida

5. nullipara

6. primigravida

7. primipara

8. multigravida

9. multipara

10. viability

11. preterm

12. term

13. postterm

14. human chorionic gonadotrophin (HCG)

15. C

16. P

17. K

18. T

19. S

20. U

21. J

22. N

23. B

24. G

25. A

26. O

27. I

28. Q

29. E

30. M

31. F

32. H

33. D

34. R

35. L

36. *Complete table related to signs and symptoms of pregnancy:* presumptive, probable, positive; see Table 9-2 for identification of signs and symptoms in each category along with time of occurrence and possible causes other than pregnancy for the categories of presumptive and probable.

37. *Use of four-digit and five-digit system of obstetrical history:*
    A. 1-1-0-1; 3-1-1-0-1
    B. 2-0-1-2; 4-2-0-1-2
    C. 1-1-1-3; 4-1-1-1-3

38. T

39. F

40. F

41. T

42. F

43. T

44. F

45. T

46. F

47. T

48. T

49. F

50. F

51. F

52. T

53. T

54. F

55. F

56. *Changes in vital signs as pregnancy progresses:*
    A. *Blood pressure and heart rate patterns:* See Box 9-3; blood pressure decreases in the second trimester by 5 to 10 mm Hg and returns to baseline during the third trimester; pulse increases by 10 to 15 BPM; murmurs and palpitations can occur. *Respiratory rate pattern:* see Box 9-4; breathing becomes more thoracic in nature and volume is deeper with a slight increase in rate. Some shortness of breath may be experienced in the second half of pregnancy as

diaphragm is pushed up by enlarging uterus until lightening occurs. *Temperature:* baseline temperature increases by about 1° Fahrenheit because of increase in BMR and effects of progesterone, secretion; woman can experience heat intolerance as a result.

57. *Mean arterial pressure:* use formula of

$$\frac{\text{systolic} + 2\,(\text{diastolic})}{3}$$

results are: 91, 81, 90, 110

58. *Specify value changes in selected laboratory tests:*
- CBC: See Box 9-3.
- Clotting activity: See Circulation and coagulation times subsection of Body Systems—Cardiopulmonary system section.
- Acid-base balance: See Box 9-6.
- Urinalysis: See Box 9-6.

59. *Expected adaptations in elimination:*
- renal: See Renal system subsection; slowed passage of urine and dilatation of ureters as a result of progesterone increases possibility of UTIs; bladder irritability, nocturia, urinary frequency and urgency (first and third trimesters after lightening).
- bowel: See Esophagus, stomach, and intestines subsection; constipation and hemorrhoids; effect of progesterone, which decreases peristalsis and intestinal displacement.

60. *Changes in endocrine function and secretions of hormones:* See Endocrine system subsection for full description of each hormone and how it changes with pregnancy.

Crossword Puzzle

Across: 1. quickening; 3. Hegars; 5. Braxton Hicks; 9. Couvade; 10. funic souffle; 13. ambivalence; 14. term; 15. epulis; 16. striae gravidarum; 18. tubercles; 20. lightening; 24. pica; 25. ptyalism; 27. amenorrhea; 28. operculum; 29. lability

Down: 2. cravings; 4. gravida; 6. chloasma; 7. Goodells; 8. leukorrhea; 11. uterine souffle; 12. Kegel; 17. Chadwicks; 19. colostrum; 21. trimester; 22. Nägeles; 23. Lamaze; 25. pyrosis; 26. parity

Critical Thinking Exercises

1. *Responses to patient concerns and questions*
   A. *Spotting after intercourse:* Discuss cervical and vaginal friability/fragility and increased vascularity; makes the vagina and cervix softer and more delicate so spotting after intercourse is expected; caution that any bleeding should be reported so it can be evaluated.
   B. *Use of a home pregnancy test:* Use Teaching Guidelines Box—Home Pregnancy Testing; emphasize the importance of following directions carefully since each brand is a little different; use first-voided morning specimen for most concentrated urine and notify health care provider for an appointment regardless of the test result.
   C. *Bladder and vaginal infections:* Discuss impact of increased vaginal secretions that are more alkaline and impact of stasis of urine that contains nutrients and has a higher pH; review prevention measures at this time (see Chapter 10).
   D. *Breast changes with pregnancy:* Discuss changes in breasts such as enlargement of Montgomery's tubercles and development of ducts, lobules, and alveolar tissue resulting in larger breasts that are tender during the first trimester. Tell patient that she may notice changes in consistency and presence of lumpiness when she does breast self-examination.
   E. *Effect of pregnant woman's position:* Discuss supine hypotensive syndrome, which is caused by compression of the vena cava and abdominal aorta when the woman is in a supine position; car-

diac output decreases and blood pressure falls; lateral position for rest is best.

F. *Nosebleeds:* Tell her estrogen increases the vascularity of the upper respiratory tract and causes edema, congestion, and hyperemia of the tissue, making nosebleeds more common.

G. *Ankle edema:* Explain that the swelling of her ankles is a result of the pressure of her enlarging uterus and the dependent position of her legs. The iliac veins and inferior vena cava increase venous pressure and decrease blood flow; elevating legs and exercising them helps to decrease edema. Caution her never to take someone else's medications or to self-medicate.

H. *Posture change and low back pain:* Lordosis occurs as a result of the enlargement of the uterus, which decreases abdominal muscle tone and increased mobility of the pelvic joints, tilting the pelvis forward. This results in lower back pain, a change in posture, and shifting forward of the center of gravity.

I. *Braxton Hicks:* The woman is describing false labor contractions since they diminish when she increases her activity level; these contractions facilitate blood flow and promote oxygen delivery to the fetus. Compare these contractions with true labor contractions (see Chapter 13).

J. *Shortness of breath during pregnancy:* Explain that what she is experiencing is a result of increased sensitivity of her respiratory center to carbon dioxide and the elevation of the diaphragm by the enlarging uterus. Assess the woman for signs of pulmonary edema to be sure the shortness of breath is physiologic rather than pathologic in nature.

2. *Blood pressure protocol:* Consider the effects of maternal age, activity level, health status, level of stress, and position; protocol should emphasize consistency in arm used and patient position, use of the proper size of cuff, provide time for the woman to relax before the blood pressure is assessed, repeat if the reading is elevated.

Chapter 10: Nursing Care During Pregnancy
Chapter Review Activities

1. presumptive, probable, positive

2. Nägele's, estimated date of birth, three months, seven days, last menstrual period, trimesters

3. Supine hypotension, pallor, dizziness, breathlessness, tachycardia, nausea, clammy skin (sweating)

4. fundal height, pinch

5. health status, fetal movement, FHR, rhythm, gestational age

6. developmental, accepting the pregnancy, identifying with the role of mother, reordering relationships with her mother and her partner, establishing a relationship with the unborn child, preparing for the birth experience

7. biological fact of pregnancy, "I am pregnant," growing fetus as distinct from herself, person to nurture, "I am going to have a baby," birth, parenting, "I am going to be a mother"

8. announcement, moratorium, focusing

9. birth plan

10. prescriptions, proscriptions, taboos

11. Down syndrome, 16 to 18, MSAFP, HCG, unconjugated estriol

12. *Pregnancy and violence:*
    A. *State harmful effects:* injury to mother and/or fetus, inadequate or late prenatal care, increased rate of LBW, anxiety, depression, low maternal weight gain, increased risk for infection and anemia, may use alcohol or drugs to cope
    B. *Target body parts:* head, breasts, abdomen, genitalia
    C. *Difficulties that may suggest battering:* inadequate diet including milk and milk products, lack of sleep, minimal forms of self-relaxation, does not take proper care of herself

13. B

14. D

15. A

16. C

17. E

18. *Calculating expected date of birth:* Use Nägele's rule by subtracting three months and adding seven days (and sometimes one year) to the first day of the last menstrual period.
    A. February 12, 1999
    B. October 21, 1997
    C. April 11, 1999

19. *Cultural beliefs and practices:* See Cultural variations subsection of Variations in prenatal care.
    A. *Describe how cultural beliefs affect participation in prenatal care:* Consider the following factors: beliefs that conflict with typical prenatal practices, lack of money and transportation, communication difficulties, concern regarding modesty and gender of health care provider, fear of invasive procedures, view of pregnancy as healthy whereas health care providers imply illness, view of pregnancy problems as a normal part of pregnancy

    B. *Proscriptions and prescriptions:* See specific subsections for emotional responses, clothing, physical activity and rest, sexual activity, dietary practices.

20. *Completing table regarding components of initial and follow-up visits:* See subsections for the Initial visit and Follow-up visits in the Care management—assessment and nursing diagnoses section.

21. *Components of fetal assessment:* measurement of fundal height, gestational age determination, health status of fetus including FHR and pattern, fetal movements, and unusual/abnormal maternal or fetal signs and symptoms; see specific subsections for each component in the Follow-up visits section.

22. *List signs of potential complications during pregnancy:* See Signs of Potential Complications Box, which lists signs according to the first, second, and third trimesters.

23. *Nursing approach when discussing signs of complications with pregnant woman and her family:*
    • discuss the signs, possible cause, when and to whom to report
    • present the signs verbally and in written form
    • provide time to answer questions and discuss concerns; make follow-up phone calls
    • gather full information of signs that are reported; use information as the basis for action
    • document all assessments, actions, and responses

24. T

25. F

26. T

27. T

28. T

29. F

30. F

31. T

32. F

33. T

34. F

35. T

36. F

37. T

38. F

39. F

40. F

41. T

42. T

43. F

44. T

45. T

46. T

47. *Protocol for fundal measurement:* Consider woman's position, type of measuring tape used (paper, non-stretchable), measurement method (Fig. 10-8), and conditions of the examination, such as an empty bladder and relaxed or contracted uterus

48. *Factors used to estimate gestational age:* menstrual history, contraceptive history, pregnancy test result, and specific findings related to the maternal-fetal unit, for example time of appearance of the specific signs of pregnancy

49. *Principles of body mechanics:* See Figs. 10-13, 10-15 and Home Care Box—Posture and Body Mechanics.

50. *Safety guidelines with rationale:* See Teaching Guidelines Box—Safety During Pregnancy and the prevention measures identified in each subsection of Education for self-care section.

51. *Contraindications for breastfeeding:* deep-seated aversion to breastfeeding by the mother or her partner, need to take certain medications that are harmful to the newborn, medical disorders such as active TB, newly diagnosed breast cancer, hepatitis C, and HIV positive status in developed countries.

Critical Thinking Exercises

1. *Health history interview:* See Initial visit subsection of Assessment and nursing diagnoses section.

   A. *Purpose of health history interview:*
      - establish a therapeutic relationship with the woman and those who come with her
      - planned time for purposeful communication to gather baseline data related to woman's subjective appraisal of her health status and to gather objective information based on nurse's observation of the woman's affect, posture, body language, skin color, and other physical and emotional signs

   B. *Components:* reason for seeking care, current pregnancy, OB/GYN history, medical history, nutritional history, drug use, family history, social and experiential history, review of systems

   C. *Write two questions for each component:* Be sure questions reflect the principles of effective questioning; consider the need to plan in follow-up questions to clarify and gather further information when a problem is identified. Each question should be clear, understandable, open-ended, and seek only one piece of information.

2. *Care of woman at initial visit who is anxious and unsure about prenatal care:* answer should emphasize
   - establishing a therapeutic, trusting relationship that will make the woman comfortable about coming for further prenatal care
   - teaching the patient about the importance of prenatal care for her own health and that of her baby
   - involving her boyfriend in the care process so he will encourage her participation in prenatal care
   - following guidelines for health history interview, physical examination, and laboratory tests; ensuring her privacy and comfort during the examination and teaching her about how her body is changing
   - evaluating desire for this pregnancy and the need for community agency support

3. *Couple during the first trimester:* concerns and questions
   A. *Accuracy of EDB:* Reliability depends on the accuracy of the date of first day of her LMP and the regularity of her menstrual cycles; birth can normally occur one to two weeks before or after the calculated EDB.
   B. *Kegel exercises:* pelvic muscle exercises to maintain muscle tone and ability to support organs; see Kegel exercises subsection of Education for self-care section and Teaching Guidelines Box— Kegel Exercises (Chapter 4).
   C. *Effect of pregnancy on sexuality:* See Home Care Box—Sexuality in Pregnancy; emphasize that intercourse is safe as long as pregnancy is progressing in a healthy manner; sexual expression should be in tune with the woman's changing needs and emotions. Inform

couple that spotting can occur afterward because of cervical and vaginal changes with pregnancy and that changes in positions and activities may be helpful as pregnancy progresses.
   D. *Morning sickness:* See Table 10-2 (first trimester section); fully assess what she is experiencing, then discuss why it happens, how long it will last, and relief measures.

4. *Physical activity and exercise in pregnancy:* See Physical activity subsection of the Education for self-care section and Home Care Box—Exercise Tips for Pregnant Woman; assess her usual exercise patterns and consider their safety; discuss precautions and guidelines for safe, effective exercise; emphasize that moderate physical activity benefits her and her baby and will prepare her for the work of labor and birth.

5. *Nursing diagnosis, expected outcome, and nursing measures for pregnant women in various situations:*
   A. Risk for urinary tract infection related to lack of knowledge regarding changes in renal system during pregnancy. Woman will drink at least three liters of fluid each day and empty bladder at first urge. Nursing measures: increase fluid intake, use acid ash-forming fluids such as cranberry juice, void frequently, perform adequate perineal hygiene, use side lying position when resting to enhance renal perfusion and urine formation.
   B. Pain in lower back related to neuromuscular changes associated with pregnancy at 23 weeks gestation; woman will experience lessening of lower back pain following implementation of suggested relief measures; nursing measures should include explanation of the basis for lower back pain and relief measures including back rubs, pelvic

rock, and posture changes (see Table 10-2). In addition, encourage woman to change her footwear for better stability and safety.

C. Moderate anxiety related to lack of knowledge concerning the process of labor and birth and appropriate measures to cope with the pain and discomfort. Couple will enroll in childbirth classes in the seventh month of pregnancy. Nursing measure should include overview of childbirth process and current measures, both nonpharmacologic and pharmacologic, used to relieve pain and role of the coach. Nurse should make a referral to childbirth classes, assist with preparation of birth plan, and discuss childbirth options and pre-birth preparations.

6. *Formulation of a birth plan:* See Birth plan subsection of Options for childbearing families section.
   A. *Describe:* Plan should include partner's role during childbirth, who will be coach and who will be present, setting for the birth, labor management measures including anesthesia, comfort measures, position during labor and birth, events at the birth, newborn and postpartum care.
   B. *Purpose:* means of open communication about the childbirth process between the woman and her partner and between the couple and their health care providers
   C. *Nurse's approach in formulation of a birth plan:* Begin discussion early in pregnancy so full consideration can be given to each option, identify components that should be included, and facilitate decision-making concerning options

7. *Woman in the second trimester:* questions and concerns
   A. *Purpose of fundal height measurement:* indirect assessment of her fetus' growth

B. *Determination of fetal health status:* Discuss assessment measures including fundal height, FHR and pattern, and fetal movement; teach her how to assess her baby's movements starting in the third trimester and let her listen to the baby's heartbeat.
   C. *Clothing choice during pregnancy:* Consider safety and comfort in terms of wearing low-heeled shoes and nonrestrictive clothing including leg coverings.
   D. *Gas and constipation:* See Table 10-2 (Second trimester section); assess problem and lifestyle; suggest fluids, roughage, activity as relief measures.
   E. *Itchiness:* If woman seems to be experiencing noninflammatory pruritus, make sure there are no unusual rashes indicating a possible reaction to a medication or substance. Use Table 10-2 (Second trimester section) for basis of the discomfort and relief measures.
   F. *Travel during pregnancy:* See Travel subsection of Self-care section. Tell her that she may travel if her pregnancy is progressing normally; emphasize importance of staying hydrated, wearing seat belt, doing breathing and foot/ankle/leg exercises, ambulating every hour for 15 minutes, and voiding every two hours.

8. Supine hypotension syndrome: See Emergency Box—Supine Hypotension.
   A. *Explanation of assessment findings:* . supine hypotension
   B. *Immediate action:* Turn on side and keep her in this position until vital signs stabilize and signs and symptoms diminish.

9. Woman in the third trimester: questions and concerns
   A. *Nipple condition for breastfeeding:* Perform pinch test to see if nipples will evert; if they do not the woman can use

a nipple shell inside her bra to help the nipples protrude. No special exercises are recommended since they could stimulate preterm labor in susceptible women; keep nipples and areola clean.

B. *Ankle edema:* See Table 10-2 (Third trimester section). Discuss basis for the edema and encourage use of leg/ankle/foot exercises and elevating legs periodically during the day (Fig. 10-16); emphasize importance of fluid intake.

C. *Leg cramps:* See Table 10-2 (Third trimester section) and Fig. 10-19. Discuss cause then demonstrate relief measures such as pressing weight onto the foot while standing or dorsiflexing the foot while lying in bed; avoid pointing the toes.

10. Concerns about preterm labor and birth
    A. *Signs of preterm labor:* See Home Care Box—How to Recognize Preterm Labor and Fig. 10-20.
    B. *Action if signs are noted:* Empty bladder, drink three to four glasses of water, lie on side and continue to assess contractions for one more hour; if contractions do not diminish, notify the primary health care provider.

11. *Sibling preparation:* To formulate answer use Sibling adaptation subsection of Preparing for childbirth section and Box 10-1, which provides tips for sibling preparation. Emphasize importance of considering each child's developmental level; prepare children for prenatal events, time during hospitalization, and the homecoming of the new baby; refer to sibling classes and encourage sibling visitation after birth.

12. *Woman experiencing emotional lability:* See Maternal adaptation section and Table 10-2 (First trimester section); discuss hormonal basis of mood swings and experiences during the first trimester including ambivalence; identify measures her husband can use to help.

13. *Woman exhibiting introspection:* See Reordering personal relationships subsection. Explain that she is concentrating on having a baby and forming a relationship with her fetus; emphasize her partner's role as caregiver and nurturer.

14. *Home birth:* See Home birth subsection of Options for childbearing families. Answer should include home preparation including obtaining supplies and equipment, arranging for medical backup and transportation in the event of an emergency, and choosing and preparing those attending the birth.

Chapter 11: Maternal and Fetal Nutrition
Chapter Review Activities

1. intrauterine growth restriction, low birth weight, preterm, small for gestational age, small for gestational age, preterm

2. age, activity level, current weight, number of fetuses, alteration in health, energy, 300 Kcal

3. pregnant adolescents, poor women, women who adhere to unusual diets

4. iron deficiency anemia, adolescents, African-Americans

5. Lactose intolerance

6. Pica, clay, laundry starch, corn starch, ice, food cravings

7. OB/GYN effects on nutrition, medical history, usual maternal diet, anthropometric measurements, height, weight, body mass index (BMI)

8. vegetables, fruits, legumes, nuts, seeds, grains, semivegetarian, lactoovovegetarians, vegans, strict vegetarians

9. Pyrosis

10. *Complete nutrient table:* Use Table 11-1 and specific subsections for each nutrient.

11. *Indicators of nutritional risks:* See Box 11-1.

12. *Guidelines to follow when planning menu with a vegan:* See Vegetarian diets subsection of Plan of care and interventions section. Consider that this woman's diet is deficient in B_{12} (needs supplementation) and low in iron, calcium, zinc, B_6, and perhaps calories; food needs to be combined to ensure that all amino acids are provided.

13. *Signs of good and poor nutrition:* See Table 11-3 for full list of signs in terms of specific body functions and areas.

14. *Nursing measures for specific nursing diagnoses:* See appropriate subsection in Coping with nutrition-related discomforts of pregnancy section.
    A. *Altered nutrition: less than body's requirements related to inadequate intake associated with nausea and vomiting:* See Box 11-5 for a food plan and Nausea and vomiting subsection for identification of relief measures.
    B. *Altered elimination: constipation related to decreased intestinal motility associated with increased progesterone level during pregnancy:* See Constipation subsection; measures include fluid and roughage intake, exercise/activity, and regular time for elimination.

15. *Calculation of BMI and determination of weight gain pattern:* Use Fig. 11-3 to calculate BMI and Box 11-4 to determine weight gain pattern based on a woman's BMI; all women should gain approximately 1–2.5 kg in the first trimester; weight gain per week is recommended for the second and third trimester.

June: BMI 21, normal; total 11.5 to 16 kg; 0.4 kg/week
Alice: BMI 33, obese; total at least 7 kg; 0.3 kg/week
Ann: BMI 16, underweight; total 12.5 to 18 kg; 0.5 kg/week

16. T

17. F

18. T

19. T

20. F

21. T

22. T

23. F

24. T

25. F

26. T

27. F

28. T

29. F

30. F

31. T

32. T

33. T

34. *Nutrition guidelines for lactation:* adequate calcium intake, at least 1800 Kcal/day, adequate fluid intake, and avoiding tobacco, alcohol, and excessive caffeine

35. *Factors that increase nutrient need during pregnancy:* growth and development of

uterine placental fetal unit, expansion of maternal blood volume and RBCs, mammary changes, increased BMR

Critical Thinking Exercises

1. *Nutrition and weight gain concerns*
   A. *Concern regarding amount of recommended weight gain:*
      - identify components of maternal weight gain; use Fig. 11-5 to illustrate how the weight gain is distributed
      - discuss impact of maternal weight gain on fetal growth and development; association between poor maternal weight gain and low birth weight and infant mortality
      - discuss weight gain total and pattern for a woman with a normal 19.5 BMI
   B. *Eating for two during pregnancy:*
      - emphasis on quality food that meets nutritional requirements, not on the quantity of food
      - discuss expected weight gain total and pattern for a normal 21.5 BMI; appropriate nutrient intake will reflect this pattern
      - excessive weight gain during pregnancy may be difficult to lose after and could lead to chronic obesity
   C. *Vitamin supplementation during pregnancy:* Determine what and how much she takes; compare to recommendations for pregnancy; discuss potential problems with toxicity, especially with overuse of fat-soluble vitamins.
   D. *Heartburn:* Recommend relief measures: small, frequent meals; fluid between and not with meals; avoid spicy, fatty foods; stay upright after meals
   E. *Weight reduction diets during pregnancy:*
      - BMI indicates overweight status; she should gain approximately 7 to 11.5 kg during pregnancy

   - discuss hazards of inadequate caloric intake during pregnancy in terms of growth and development of fetus (LBW) and pregnancy-related structures; impact of ketoacidosis
   - discuss quality foods and the development of good nutritional habits to be used during the postpartum period as part of a sensible weight reduction plan
   - discuss importance of exercise and activity during pregnancy
   F. *Reduction of water intake:* Discuss importance of fluid to meet demands of pregnancy-related changes, regulate temperature, prevent constipation and UTIs; consider possible association between preterm labor and dehydration.
   G. *Lactose intolerance:* Discuss basis for problem; reduce lactose intake by using nondairy calcium sources and calcium supplements; take Lactase supplements.
   H. *Weight loss with lactation:* Discuss weight loss patterns with lactation; emphasize that fat store from pregnancy is used during the lactation process with a resultant weight loss; inform her of increased need for nutrients, calories and fluids, which are used up in the process of lactation.

2. *Taking iron supplements effectively:* See Iron subsection of Nutrient needs section, Iron supplementation subsection of Plan of care and interventions, Table 11-1 for iron sources, and Home Care Box—Iron Supplementation
   - discuss importance of iron
   - emphasize importance of vitamin C for iron absorption; discuss food sources for both vitamin C and iron
   - discuss ways to take iron supplements to enhance absorption and minimize side effects including GI upset and constipation

3. *Native American woman—meeting nutritional needs*
    A. *Counseling approach:*
        - assess her current nutritional status and habits; obtain a diet history
        - analyze current patterns as a basis for menu planning
        - discuss weight gain pattern for an underweight woman
        - use a variety of teaching methods; keep woman actively involved
        - emphasize importance of good nutrition for herself and her newborn
    B. *Menu plan:* Use Table 11-4 for specific Native American-type foods, and Table 11-2 to determine number of servings of required nutrients when planning the one day menu; be sure to distribute nutrients throughout the day in meals and snacks

Chapter 12: Factors and Processes of Labor and Birth

Chapter Review Activities

1. membrane-filled spaces, sutures, intersect

2. overlapping, bones of the fetal skull

3. part of the fetus, pelvic inlet, cephalic, breech, shoulder

4. first felt by the examiner's finger, vaginal examination, occiput, sacrum, scapula

5. fully flexed, occiput

6. long axis (spine) of the fetus to the long axis (spine) of the mother, spines are parallel, spines are at right angles (perpendicular)

7. fetal body parts to each other, general flexion

8. largest transverse diameter, smallest anteroposterior diameter, flexion

9. fetal presenting part, four quadrants of the maternal pelvis

10. largest transverse diameter, maternal pelvic brim or inlet into the true pelvis, ischial spines

11. presenting part, maternal ischial spines, centimeters, ischial spines, descent

12. shortening and thinning, cervix, first, percentages

13. enlargement, widening, cervical os, cervical canal, centimeters, 1 to 10

14. fetal presenting part (usually the head) descends (drops), true pelvis, two weeks, onset of true labor

15. brownish or blood-tinged, mucus plug, ripens

16. turns and adjustments, fetal head, maternal bony pelvis, cardinal movements, engagement, descent, flexion, internal rotation, extension, external rotation and restitution, expulsion (birth)

17. Valsalva maneuver, intrathoracic pressure, venous return, venous pressure, hypoxia

18. *Identify/describe five factors affecting progress of labor:* See separate subsection for each of the five factors, namely passenger, passageway, powers, position of mother, psychologic response of mother.

19. *Events of the four states of labor:* See Stages of labor subsection of the Process of labor section
    first: cervical stage with effacement and dilatation
    second: birth stage with birth of fetus
    third: placental stage with separation and expulsion of the placenta
    fourth: recovery stage with maternal stabilization after birth

20. *Describe the cardinal movements of labor:*
See Mechanism of labor subsection in the Process of labor section and Fig. 12-14; engagement and descent, flexion, internal rotation, extension, external rotation and restitution, expulsion.

21. *Label illustrations:*
Fetal skull: A, mentum (chin); B, occipitofrontal diameter; C, frontal bone (sinciput); D, suboccipitobregmatic diameter; E, parietal bone (vertex); F, occipitomental diameter; G, occiput; H, sagittal suture; I, lambdoid suture; J, posterior fontanel; K, biparietal diameter; L, coronal suture; M, frontal suture and bone; N, anterior fontanel (bregma)

Maternal pelvis: A, symphysis pubis; B, anteroposterior diameter; C, transverse diameter; D, sacral promontory; E, sacrum; F, sacroiliac joint; G, ischial spine; H, pubic bone; I, sacrotuberous ligament; J, pubic arch; K, ischial tuberosity; L, coccyx; M, sacroiliac joint

22. *Presentation, presenting part, position, lie, and attitude for each illustration:*
A. cephalic, occiput, LOA, longitudinal, flexion
B. cephalic, occiput, LOT, longitudinal, flexion
C. cephalic, occiput, LOP, longitudinal, flexion
D. cephalic, occiput, ROA, longitudinal, flexion
E. cephalic, occiput, ROT, longitudinal, flexion
F. cephalic, occiput, ROP, longitudinal, flexion
G. cephalic, mentum, LMA, longitudinal, extension
H. cephalic, mentum, RMP, longitudinal, extension
I. cephalic, mentum, RMA, longitudinal, extension
J. breech, sacrum, LSA, longitudinal, flexion
K. breech, sacrum, LSP, longitudinal, flexion
L. shoulder, scapula, ScA, transverse, flexion

23. *Factors that affect fetal circulation:*
   • maternal position, blood pressure, cardiac output
   • uterine contractions
   • umbilical cord blood flow

24. F

25. T

26. F

27. F

28. T

29. T

30. F

31. T

32. F

33. F

34. T

35. F

36. F

37. T

Crossword puzzle

Across: 2. first; 4. extension; 5. placental; 7. ischial spines; 9. molding; 12. lightening; 14. occiput; 16. presentation; 18. suboccipitobregmatic; 20. attitude; 21. ripening; 22. posterior; 24. bregma; 25. efface; 27. prodromal; 30. pushing; 31. bony pelvis; 33. lie; 34. internal; 35. frequency; 36. dilate; 37. intensity; 38. duration

Down: 1. external; 3. second; 6. bloody; 8. station; 9. mentum; 10. fourth; 11. cephalic;

13. gynecoid; 15. partogram; 17. restitution;
19. sacrum; 22. primary powers; 23. breech;
26. flexion; 27. position; 28. sagittal;
29. descent; 32. engaged

Critical Thinking Exercises

1. *Analysis of vaginal examination:*

   Exam I: ROP (right occiput posterior, cephalic [vertex] presentation, longitudinal lie, flexed attitude), −1 (station at one centimeter above the ischial spines), 50 percent effaced, 3 cm dilated

   Exam II: RMA (right mentum anterior, cephalic [face] presentation, longitudinal lie, extended attitude), 0 (station at the ischial spines), 25 percent effaced, 2 cm dilated

   Exam III: LST (left sacrum transverse, breech presentation, longitudinal lie, flexed attitude), +1 (station at 1 cm below the ischial spines), 75 percent effaced, 6 cm dilated

   Exam IV: OA (occiput anterior, cephalic (vertex) presentation, longitudinal lie, flexed attitude), +3 (station at 3 cm below the ischial spines near or on the perineum), 100 percent (fully effaced), and 10 cm (fully dilated)

2. *Woman with questions/concerns regarding the process of labor:*

   A. *Onset of labor:* See Onset of labor subsection of the Process of labor section; interaction of fetal and maternal hormonal changes, uterine distension, aging of placenta, oncofetal fibronectin.

   B. *Signs of prodromal labor:* See Box 12-1, in which signs preceding labor are identified including lightening, urinary frequency, backache, Braxton Hicks contractions, weight loss, energy surge, bloody show, possible rupture of the membranes. Health care provider would note cervical changes in terms of ripening, dilatation, and effacement.

   C. *Duration of labor:* see Stages of labor subsection for approximate times; give woman ranges but not absolutes (espe-
      cially since this will be her first labor); discuss her role in facilitating the progress of labor.

   D. *Position changes during labor:*
      - emphasize that the position of the woman is one of the five Ps of labor
      - discuss each position and describe its effect (Fig. 12-12)
      - demonstrate each position and have her practice them with her partner
      - emphasize beneficial effects of ambulation and changing positions on fetus, circulation, comfort, and progress

Chapter 13: Management of Discomfort

Chapter Review Activities

1. Visceral, cervical, ischemia, lower portion, lumbar area, thighs

2. Somatic, perineal, perineal tissue, peritoneum, uterocervical support

3. Referred, back, flank, thighs

4. gate control, massage, stroking, music, imagery, concentrating on breathing techniques

5. Endorphins

6. Dick-Read, Lamaze, Bradley

7. Dick-Read, fear of the unknown, understanding, confidence, labor and birth, nutrition, hygiene, exercise, physical exercise, conscious relaxation, breathing patterns, deep abdomen, shallow breathing

8. Lamaze, conditioned response, controlled muscular relaxation, breathing patterns, chest breathing, intensity of uterine contractions, progress of labor, concentrating on a focal point, painful stimuli, partner, monitrice

9. Bradley, harmony with the body, breath control, abdominal breathing, general body relaxation, darkness, solitude, quiet

10. walk, talk, slow abdominal, half

11. more shallow, twice

12. cleansing breath

13. transition, hyperventilation, respiratory alkalosis, lightheadedness, dizziness, tingling of fingers, circumoral numbness, breathe into a paper bag or cupped hand, carbon dioxide

14. Effleurage, counterpressure, gate control

15. Water therapy, active, 36.7° C, 37.8° C, temperature, FHR

16. Transcutaneous electrical stimulation (TENS), placebo, endogenous opiates

17. *Factors influencing response to pain:* culture, anxiety/fear, previous experience with pain and childbirth, support, history of substance abuse, history of sexual abuse, pain tolerance and perception

18. *Theoretic basis of effectiveness of massage, stroking, music, and imagery in reducing pain sensation:* Discuss the gate control theory of pain; see Factors influencing pain response section.

19. B

20. F

21. H

22. A

23. G

24. J

25. D

26. I

27. L

28. C

29. E

30. K

31. *Complete table related to types of regional anesthetics:* See appropriate subsections for local infiltration, pudendal block, spinal block, and epidural block in the Pharmacologic management of discomfort section.

32. *Systemic analgesics:* See Systemic analgesia subsection of Pharmacologic management of discomfort.
    A. *Factors influencing effect of systemic analgesics on fetus:* maternal dosage, pharmacokinetics of the specific drug, route, time when administered during labor
    B. *Fetal effects systemic analgesics:* central nervous system depression as a result of the direct effect of the drug when it crosses the placenta and/or the indirect effect of maternal hypotension and hypoventilation resulting from the drug's action on maternal function; CNS depression slows the FHR and decreases variability, and leads to respiratory depression and hypoxia.

33. *Examples of narcotic analgesic, mixed narcotic agonist-antagonist compound, analgesic potentiator, and narcotic antagonist and how each is used in childbirth:* See Table 13-1 and specific subsections for each classification in Pharmacologic management of discomfort section.

34. T

35. F

36. T

37. T

38. F

39. T

40. F

41. T

42. T

43. F

44. T

45. F

46. T

47. T

Critical Thinking Exercises

1. *Explaining the basis of childbirth pain to expectant fathers:* Explain the neurologic origins of pain (see subsection in Discomfort during labor section); describe how women experience the pain and factors that influence the experience; discuss measures to help the woman reduce and cope with the pain.

2. *Nurse sensitivity to patient pain experience* (see Expression of pain subsection of Discomfort during labor section and Nonpharmacologic management of discomfort section)
   A. *Signs and expressions of pain in labor:*
      Physical signs: alteration in vital signs, skin color, diaphoresis, vomiting
      Affective expressions: anxiety, writhing, crying, groaning, gesturing, muscular movements
   B. *Measures nurses can use to alter perception of pain:* Consider the specific factors influencing each woman's response when determining measures.

3. *Working with a couple with unrealistic, inaccurate views regarding pain and pain relief during labor:* See Care management section.
   - inform couple regarding basis of pain and its potentially adverse effects on the maternal-fetal unit and the progress of labor; pain can inhibit labor as a result of the stress response, and circulation can be altered
   - discuss a variety of nonpharmacologic and pharmacologic measures and their effects, including level of safety, benefit for the maternal-fetal unit, and ability to enhance the progress of labor
   - emphasize that mother and fetus will be thoroughly assessed before, during, and after any measure

4. *Benefits of water therapy:*
   - describe the beneficial effects of water therapy and how it can facilitate the labor process by promoting relaxation and relief of discomfort and tension, and shortening the duration of labor, thereby decreasing the possibility of cesarean birth; use research findings to substantiate these claims
   - describe the successful experiences of other clinical agencies implementing water therapy and how this has affected the number of births per year
   - use the favorable reports of women who have used water therapy; consider how this could affect what they tell other women of childbearing age

5. *Occurrence of hypotension after administration of epidural during labor (see Emergency Box—Maternal Hypotension with Decreased Placental Perfusion)*
   A. *What is being experienced by this woman:* Maternal hypotension decreases placental perfusion and results in an alteration in fetal oxygen level, reflected in the change in FHR and variability.
   B. *Immediate nursing actions:* Turn woman on side or put wedge under hip, maintain IV infusion, administer

oxygen, elevate legs, assess maternal-fetal unit for effectiveness of actions taken; notify primary health-care provider for further instructions.

6. *Woman receiving an epidural block:* See Epidural block subsection of Pharmacologic management of discomfort section.
   A. *Assessment prior to induction of block:* status of maternal-fetal unit, progress of labor in terms of phase, contraindications to use
   B. *Preparation measures:* Answer should reflect actions related to explanation, consent, hydration, bladder condition.
   C. *Positions for induction:* lateral (modified Sims') or sitting with back curved to separate vertebrae; assist her with positioning and maintaining position without movement during the induction
   D. *Nursing management during the epidural block:* Assess response on maternal-fetal unit and progress of labor, maintain hydration, assist with bladder emptying and positioning of legs safely, change position frequently, maintain site to prevent infection; consider anesthesia recovery in the postpartum period.

Chapter 14: Fetal Monitoring

Chapter Review Activities

1. reassuring, nonreassuring, compromised, hypoxemia, hypoxia

2. auscultation, fetoscope, ultrasound device

3. Electronic fetal monitoring, ultrasound transducer, tocotransducer, spiral electrode, intrauterine pressure catheter

4. Oligohydramnios, variable deceleration, amnioinfusion

5. *Factors that affect fetal oxygen supply and expected characteristics of FHR and uterine activity* (see Fetal response subsection in Basis for monitoring section)
   A. *Factors that can reduce fetal oxygen supply:* reduction in blood flow through maternal vessels, reduction in oxygen content of maternal blood, alterations in fetal circulation, and reduction in blood flow in placenta
   B. *Characteristics of reassuring FHR pattern:* baseline 110 to 160 BPM, no periodic changes, moderate baseline variability, early decelerations, accelerations with fetal movement
   C. *Characteristics of normal uterine activity:* frequency of contractions every two to five minutes, duration <90 seconds, intensity <100 mm Hg, rest period of at least 30 seconds with average IUP of 15 mm Hg or less

5. *Characteristics of nonreassuring FHR patterns:* See Fetal compromise subsection of Basis for monitoring section; characteristics are fully identified in terms of changes in rate, variability, and pattern associated with uterine contractions.

6. I

7. J

8. H

9. G

10. K

11. F

12. C

13. B

14. D

15. E

16. A

17. L

18. *Criteria to determine if FHR pattern is reassuring or nonreassuring:* Use the criteria listed in Box 14-1.

19. 20

20. 60 minutes, 30 minutes, 15 minutes

21. 30 minutes, 15 minutes, 5 minutes

22. *Intermittent auscultation to assess fetus during labor:*
    Advantages: high touch/low tech approach, natural method that facilitates activity, comfortable and noninvasive
    Disadvantages: inconvenient, time-consuming, increased anxiety of patient if nurse has difficulty locating PMI, less information is determined about the FHR pattern

23. *Outline guidelines to follow for intermittent auscultation:* See Intermittent auscultation subsection of Monitoring techniques section; six specific guidelines/steps are described.

24. *Legal responsibilities related to fetal monitoring during childbirth:* See Legal Tip—Fetal Monitoring Standards in Plan of care and interventions section. Consider correct interpretation of FHR pattern as reassuring or nonreassuring, take appropriate action, evaluate response, notify primary health-care provider in a timely fashion, know the chain of command if a dispute in interpretation occurs, document assessment findings, action, and response.

25. T

26. F

27. T

28. F

29. T

30. T

31. T

32. F

33. F

34. T

35. T

36. T

37. F

38. T

39. *Emergency measures for nonreassuring patterns:* See Box 14-3—Protocol for FHR Monitoring.

40. *Nursing measures for monitored woman and family:* See Box 14-3 for detailed outline related to teaching, assessing, and caring for the monitored woman and her family during labor.

41. *Documentation regarding fetal status on patient record and monitor strip:* See Box 14-3—Protocol for Fetal Heart Rate Monitoring for identification of information that should be included in each area.

Critical Thinking Exercises

1. *Woman concerned about use of external monitoring to assess her fetus and labor:* See Box 14-4 for care measures related to fetal monitoring.
   * discuss how fetus responds to labor and how the monitor will assess these responses
   * explain the advantages and purpose of monitoring
   * show her a monitor strip and explain what it reveals; tell her how she can use the strip to help with her breathing techniques

2. *Woman whose labor is being induced and external monitoring is being used* (use Table 14-5 and Fig. 14-7, *B* to formulate answer)
   A. *Pattern described and causative factors:* late deceleration patterns are occurring as a result of uteroplacental insufficiency associated with intense uterine contractions, supine position, and placental changes (aging) resulting from post-term gestation.
   B. *Nursing interventions:* should include discontinuing induction, changing to lateral position, administering oxygen via mask, assessing response, and notifying primary health care provider. Document assessment findings, action, and response.

3. *Analysis of monitor tracings:*
   A. Reassuring FHR pattern: See Fetal response subsection in Basis for monitoring section; compare criteria of reassuring FHR pattern and normal uterine contractions with the monitor tracing.
   B. Late deceleration pattern with minimal variability: Use Figs. 14-7*B* and 14-5 and Tables 14-3 and 14-5.
   C. Bradycardia with minimal variability, average FHR of 90 BPM: Use Fig. 14-5 and Tables 14-2 and 14-3.
   D. Early deceleration: Recognize this as a reassuring pattern; use Fig. 14-7*A* and Table 14-4.
   E. Tachycardia with average rate of 210: Use Table 14-2.
   F. Variable deceleration pattern: Use Table 14-5 and Fig. 14-7*C*.

Chapter 15: Nursing Care During Labor and Birth
Chapter Review Activities
1. TL

2. FL

3. FL

4. TL

5. TL

6. FL

7. TL

8. FL

9. TL

10. TL

11. TL

12. regular contractions, cervical dilatation, effacement, mucous plug (operculum)

13. 0 cm, 3 cm, 6, 8, 4 cm, 7 cm, 3, 6, 20 to 40 minutes, 8 cm, 10 cm

14. fetus is born, cervical dilatation, effacement, baby's birth, latent, descent, transition, 57 minutes, 14 minutes, 2 hours, $1\frac{1}{2}$ hours

15. baby is born, placenta is delivered, separation, firmly contracted fundus, discoid, globular, gush of dark blood, lengthening of the cord, vaginal fullness

16. G

17. H

18. K

19. I

20. F

21. B

22. N

23. A

24. E

25. L

26. O

27. D

28. C

29. J

30. M

31. uterine contractions

32. increment

33. acme

34. decrement

35. frequency

36. intensity

37. duration

38. resting tone

39. interval

40. bearing down

41. *Assessment of uterine contractions:*
   A. *Label illustration:* A, beginning of a contraction; B, duration; C, frequency; D, relaxation (interval between contractions); E, intensity; 1, increment; 2, acme; 3, decrement
   B. *Method of assessment:* Place hand on fundus and determine changes in tone for several contractions and rest periods; press finger into fundus at peak of contraction to determine intensity.

42. *Admission of woman in labor:* See Assessment and nursing diagnosis subsection of Care management—first stage of labor section.
   A. *Information from prenatal record:* See Prenatal data subsection. Include such information as age, weight gain, health status and medical problems during pregnancy, past/present obstetric history (gravida, para) including outcomes and problems, laboratory and diagnostic testing with results, EDB, baseline data from pregnancy including VS, lab values, FHR.
   B. *Information regarding status of labor:* factors distinguishing false labor from true labor, uterine contractions (onset, characteristics), show, status of membranes, fetal movement, discomfort (location, characteristics), any other accompanying signs and symptoms since onset of labor
   C. *Information regarding current health status:* health problems, respiratory status, allergies, character and time of last oral intake, emotional status

43. F

44. F

45. T

46. F

47. T

48. F

49. T

50. T

51. T

52. T

53. F

54. F

55. F

56. F

57. T

58. F

59. F

60. F

61. T

62. *Complete table related to labor stressors and support measures:* Stressors are described in Stress in labor subsection of Assessment and nursing diagnoses—first stage of labor section; see Support measures, The father or partner during labor, Culture, and Father participation subsections in Plan of care and interventions—first stage of labor section; use Table 15-4 and Care paths for low-risk woman during the first stage of labor and the second and third stages of labor.

63. *Signs of potential complications:* See Signs of Potential Complications Box—Labor for full list to consider.

64. *Psychosocial factors to observe:* See Psychosocial factors subsection. Answer should include factors related to verbal interactions, body language, perceptual ability, discomfort level, signs indicative of abuse.

65. *Complete table related to labor positions:* See Box 15-5 and Ambulation and positioning subsection of Plan of care and interventions—first stage of labor section.

66. *Critical factors to include in physical assessment of maternal-fetal unit during labor:* See Care paths for low-risk woman in first stage of labor and second/third stages of labor.
maternal factors: VS, uterine activity, cervical changes, show/bleeding, behavior, appearance, mood, energy level, bearing down effort
fetal factors: FHR pattern, activity level, cardinal movements of labor, Apgar score

67. *Laboratory and diagnostic tests during labor:* See Laboratory and diagnostic tests subsection of Assessment and nursing diagnoses—first stage of labor section; CBC, type and Rh, analysis of urine, dipstick for protein, ketone, glucose, nitrazine and ferning tests of amniotic fluid.

68. *Complete table regarding events/behavior support measures during the second stage of labor:* Use Table 15-6.

69. *Signs indicating onset of second stage of labor:* See Assessment and nursing diagnoses section for full list of signs. Definitive sign is inability to feel the cervix, which indicates full dilatation and complete effacement.

70. *Factors influencing duration of second stage of labor:* use of regional anesthesia such as epidural block, quality of bearing down efforts and positions used, parity, size, presentation and position of the fetus, maternal pelvic adequacy, physical status of the mother including level of energy

71. *Recommended positions for second stage of labor and bearing down efforts:* See Maternal position subsection of Plan of care and interventions—prebirth considerations section and Figs. 15-16, 15-17, 15-18; describe squatting, side lying, semisitting, standing, hands and knees.

Critical Thinking Exercises

1. *Woman, thinking she is in labor, calls nurse* (see Teaching Guidelines Box—How to Distinguish True Labor from False Labor and Box 15-1)
   A. *Nursing approach:* Determine the status of her labor by asking her to describe what she is experiencing and comparing her description to the characteristics of false and true labor.
   B. *Write questions:* Questions should be clear, concise, open-ended, and directed toward distinguishing her labor status and creating a basis for action.

C. *Instructions for home care of woman in latent labor:* Discuss comfort measures, distracting activities, measures to reduce anxiety, and measures to enhance labor progress; inform regarding assessment measures to determine progress and signs of problems, when and whom to call, and when to come to the hospital; nurse can make follow-up phone call to determine how woman is progressing.

2. *Women in first stage of labor at various phases:*
   A. *Identify phase of labor for each woman:* Use Table 15-2 to determine phase: Denise: active phase; Teresa: transition; Danielle: latent.
   B. *Describe behavior and appearance expected for each woman:* Use Tables 15-2 and 15-4 for descriptions; consider the phase of the woman's labor when formulating answer.
   C. *Specify physical and emotional care required:* Use Care path—low-risk woman in first stage of labor and Table 15-4 for care measures required for each woman according to her phase of labor.

3. *Procedure for locating PMI prior to auscultation of FHR or application of ultrasound transducer:* Use Procedure Box—Leopold's Maneuvers. Realize that fetal presentation and position affect location of PMI of FHR (see Fig. 15-6) and that Leopold's maneuvers will facilitate location of this point; also realize that this point will change as the baby progresses through the birth canal.

4. *Woman in labor who experiences difficulty with vaginal examinations:* See Vaginal examination subsection of Physical examination section.
   A. *Nurse's response to woman's concern:* Explain purpose of vaginal examinations and the information obtained during each examination in terms of the progress of labor and the status of the fetus; compare the findings from a vaginal examination with the information obtained from the monitor tracing.
   B. *Measures to enhance comfort and safety:* Measures to enhance comfort include deep breathing, gentleness, limit frequency, explanation of what you are doing and the results, acknowledgment of her feelings, privacy. Safety measures include infection control (and never do if actively bleeding).

5. *Actions and rationale when membranes rupture:* immediate assessment of FHR and pattern, vaginal examination (status of cervix, check for cord prolapse), assess fluid (amount, characteristics); strict infection control measures after rupture since risk for infection increases

6. *Nursing diagnosis:* Anxiety related to lack of knowledge and experience regarding the process of childbirth
   Expected outcome: Couple will cooperate with measures to enhance progress of her labor as their anxiety level decreases
   Nursing measures: Provide full, simple explanations about each aspect of labor and care measures as they occur, demonstrate and assist with simple breathing and relaxation techniques, make use of phases of labor to tailor health teaching (doing more during latent phase and less as labor progresses), model coaching and comfort measures father can perform.

7. *Cultural and religious beliefs and practices during labor:*
   A. *Questions to determine cultural and religious preferences:* See Callister (1995) topics for questions in Cultural factors subsection of Assessment and nursing diagnoses—first stage of labor section.
   B. *Importance of determining cultural preferences:* See Cultural Considera-

tions Box. Consider preferences so couple can act in ways that are comfortable to enhance the progress of labor and their view of health-care providers. Such an approach demonstrates respect, concern, and caring.

8. *Couple surprised by changes in approaches to facilitate the labor process:* Discuss advantages of the new approaches: internal locus of control (listening to her own body) and maternal position applying principle of gravity facilitate labor and can even shorten its duration; new bearing down efforts are safer (better oxygenation) and more effective (less tiring while applying effective force to facilitate descent); new positions enhance uteroplacental circulation. Use illustrations, models, and video to help couple learn techniques; demonstrate positions and help her to practice them.

9. *Home birth:* Use Mechanism of birth vertex presentation and Immediate assessment and care of newborn sections, along with Box 15-5 to answer all components of this exercise.
   A. *Measures to reassure and comfort:* Use eye contact, assume a relaxed, calm, and confident manner, explain what is happening and what you are going to be doing throughout the childbirth process, inform her and her husband what they need to do.
   B. *Crowning* (guideline no. 6): Break membranes, tell her to pant or blow to reduce force, use Ritgen's maneuver to deliver head without trauma to fetus or maternal soft tissues.
   C. *Actions after appearance of head* (guideline no. 7): Check for cord, support head during external rotation and restitution, and ease shoulders out one at a time, with anterior first then posterior.
   D. *Prevention of neonatal heat loss* (guideline nos. 11, 12): Dry baby, wrap up with the mother, cover head.

E. *Infection control:* Use Standard Precautions Box adapting to home setting; handwashing, clean materials, wear gloves if available.
F. *Prevention of bleeding:* Breastfeed, assess fundus and massage prn, expel clots if present once fundus is firm, assess bladder and encourage to void, allow placenta to separate naturally.
G. *Documentation* (guideline no. 20, items a–i): Include date, time, assessment of mother, fetus/newborn, family present, events, blood loss, Apgar.

10. *Criteria of effective pushing:* See Bearing down efforts subsection of Plan of care and interventions—prebirth considerations section; cleansing breaths, open glottis pushing with no breath holds longer that five to seven seconds, catch breath, strong expiratory grunt, upright position.

11. *Second stage of labor with reluctance to bear down and give birth:* See Bearing down subsection.
    A. *Reasons for reluctance:* Many are listed and can include not feeling ready to be a mother, waiting for someone to come, embarrassment about pushing and what happens during BDE, fear for self and baby, giving up, previous negative experience.
    B. *Nursing intervention:* Recognize her feelings, identify her reason for not continuing, address her concerns, and help her to continue.

12. *Are episiotomies needed?* See Perineal trauma related to childbirth section; compare episiotomies with spontaneous lacerations in terms of tissue affected, long-term sequelae, healing, discomfort; compare reasons given for performing episiotomies with what research demonstrates to be true.

13. *Siblings at childbirth:* Include research findings regarding effect of sibling partici-

pation on family and on the sibling; consider developmental readiness of child and use developmental principles to prepare him or her for the experience. Evaluate parental comfort with this option; arrange for a support person to remain with the child during the entire childbirth process.

14. *Primipara exhibiting disinterest in newborn during the fourth stage of labor:* See Family during the third stage of labor and Parent-newborn relationship subsections of Plan of care and interventions—third stage of labor.
    A. *Factors accounting for this behavior:* exhaustion, discomfort, cultural beliefs, disappointment, difficult labor and birth
    B. *Nursing measures:* continue to assess response, provide for her needs, provide time for close contact with newborn when mother is more comfortable and rested

15. *Care of parents following stillbirth:* See Families experiencing loss and grief in the Intrapartal period section. Encourage expression of feelings, refer to spiritual advisor, special agency team for loss, or parent support group as appropriate, arrange to see and hold baby as desired, help to make memories (footprint, photograph, hair, etc.).

Chapter 16: Physiologic Changes

Chapter Review Activities

1. T

2. F

3. F

4. F

5. T

6. T

7. T

8. T

9. F

10. F

11. F

12. T

13. F

14. T

15. T

16. F

17. *Assessment of bladder for distension:* See Urethra and bladder subsection of Urinary system section.
    A. *Reasons why bladder distension is more likely to occur:* birth-induced trauma to urethra and bladder, edematous urethra, increased bladder capacity, effect of conduction anesthesia, pelvic soreness, lacerations and episiotomy, increased urine production as a result of diuresis
    B. *Problems associated with bladder distention:* early: Bladder pushes uterus up and to the side, preventing uterus from firmly contracting, leading to excessive bleeding; later: Over-distension can lead to stasis of urine and UTI.

18. *Factors interfering with bowel elimination:* See Bowel evacuation subsection of Gastrointestinal section. Factors include decreased muscle tone, effect of progesterone, prelabor diarrhea, lack of oral intake and dehydration from labor, anticipated discomfort related to hemorrhoids and perineal trauma, resistance to urge to defecate.

19. *Hypovolemic shock less likely to occur in postpartum woman:* See Blood volume subsection of Cardiovascular system section. Pregnancy-induced hypervolemia allows most women to tolerate considerable blood loss during childbirth; size of maternal vascular bed decreases with delivery of placenta, stimulus for vasodilation is lost, and extravascular water stored during pregnancy is mobilized.

20. *Factors increasing risk for thromboembolism:* See Coagulation factors subsection of Blood components section. Increase in clotting factors and fibrinogen levels during pregnancy continues into the postpartum period; hypercoagulable state plus vessel damage with childbirth and decreased activity level of postpartum period increase risk.

21. *Contrast lochia and nonlochial bleeding:* Use Table 16-1.

Crossword puzzle

Across: 1. oxytocin; 3. taking hold; 6. mutuality; 8. diaphoresis; 9. letting go; 12. entrainment; 14. habituation; 15. episiotomy; 17. alba; 18. serosa; 20. afterpains; 21. claiming; 23. subinvolution; 24. prolactin; 25. en face; 28. taking in; 29. colostrum; 30. responsivity

Down: 2. orthostatic; 4. involution; 5. diastasis recti abdominis; 7. biorhythmicity; 10. diuresis; 11. lochia; 12. engorgement; 13. hemorrhoid; 16. puerperium; 19. engrossment; 20. attachment; 22. rubra; 26. autolysis; 27. depression

Critical Thinking Exercises

1. *Postpartum questions and concerns*
   A. *Afterpains:* Basis includes the fact that this woman is breastfeeding; sucking of the infant stimulates the posterior pituitary gland to secrete oxytocin for the let-down reflex, but it also stimulates the uterus to contract, creating uterine cramps for the first few days postpartum.
   B. *How long uterus will be palpable through the abdomen:* After one week, the uterus is in the true pelvis; after the ninth day it will not be palpable through the abdomen.
   C. *Stages and duration of lochia:* See Lochia subsection of Uterus section. Discuss characteristics of rubra, serosa, and alba, including color, consistency, amount, odor, and duration.
   D. *Protruding abdomen:* See Abdominal section. Enlarged uterus along with stretched abdominal muscles with diminished tone creates a still-pregnant appearance for the first few weeks after birth. By six weeks the abdominal wall will return to approximately its prepregnant state: skin will regain most of its elasticity; striae will fade but remain. Discuss exercise and a sensible weight-loss program to facilitate return of tone and diminish protrusion.
   E. *Diaphoresis and diuresis:* See Postpartal diuresis subsection of Urinary section. Discuss normalcy of these processes to rid body of fluid retained during pregnancy.
   F. *Breastfeeding as a contraceptive method:* See Pituitary hormones and ovarian function section. Emphasize that breastfeeding is not a reliable method since the return of ovulation is unpredictable and may precede menstruation; discuss appropriate contraceptive measures for a breastfeeding woman, taking care to avoid hormone-based methods until lactation is firmly established.
   G. *Lactation suppression in bottle-feeding woman:* See Nonbreastfeeding mothers subsection of Breast section. Breasts will fill with milk as estrogen and progesterone levels fall; because milk is not removed the cycle shuts down and the milk is absorbed into her circulatory system. She will need to support her breasts with a snug bra, avoid warmth on her breasts and expressing any of the milk, and use ice for comfort.

H. *Sexuality during postpartum period of breastfeeding woman:* See Vagina and perineum subsection of Reproductive system and associated structures section. Discuss role of prolactin in suppressing estrogen secretion thereby decreasing vaginal lubrication and resulting in vaginal dryness and dyspareunia, which will persist until ovulation resumes; use water-soluble lubricant.

Chapter 17: Assessment and Care During the Fourth Trimester

Chapter Review Activities

1. fourth stage of labor

2. couplet care, mother and baby care, single-room maternity care

3. oxytocic

4. uterine atony, excessive bleeding (hemorrhage)

5. sitz bath

6. afterpains (afterbirth pains)

7. fatigue

8. splanchnic engorgement, orthostatic hypotension

9. Homans' sign

10. Kegel exercises

11. engorgement

12. rubella

13. Rh-immune globulin, Kleihauer-Betke test

14. *Reasons for breastfeeding in fourth stage of labor:* takes advantage of the infant's alert state during the first period of reactivity, aids in contraction of the uterus to prevent hemorrhage, good opportunity to instruct the mother and assess breasts, facilitates the bonding/attachment process, stimulates infant's bowel so bilirubin containing meconium is passed.

15. *Measures to assist with voiding:* See Prevention of bladder distension in Plan of care and interventions section. Help her to assume an upright position on bedpan or in bathroom, listen to running water, put hands in warm water, pour water over perineum with peri bottle, stand in shower or sit in a sitz bath, put spirits of peppermint in bedpan, provide analgesics.

16. *Measures to prevent thrombophlebitis:* See Prevention of thrombophlebitis subsection of Plan of care and interventions—ambulation section. Exercise legs with active ROM of knees, ankles, feet, and toes, ambulate, wear support hose, keep well hydrated.

17. *Criteria for postanesthesia recovery:* See Postanesthesia recovery subsection of Assessment and nursing diagnoses—fourth stage of labor section.
    General anesthesia: LOC/alertness, orientation, VS, oxygen saturation of at least 95 percent, deep breaths, color, keep her on her side until fully oriented and gag reflex returns to prevent aspiration
    Epidural or spinal anesthesia: return of movement and sensation in lower extremities, decrease in numbness, tingling or prickly sensation in legs, ability to feel bladder and to void

18. *Measures for bottle-feeding mother to suppress lactation and relieve discomfort of engorgement:* See Breastfeeding promotion and lactation suppression subsection of Plan of care and implementation section; wear supportive bra or breast binder 24 hours a day for at least the first 72 hours postpartum, avoid stimulating

breasts (no warm water during shower, no infant sucking, no pumping or removal of milk), apply ice packs intermittently to relieve soreness.

19. *Two major interventions to prevent post-partum hemorrhage in early postpartum period:* See Prevention of excessive bleeding section.
    • Maintain uterine tone: massage fundus if boggy, expel clots when fundus is firm, administer oxytocic medications, breastfeed
    • Prevent bladder distension

20. T

21. F

22. T

23. T

24. F

25. F

26. T

27. F

28. F

29. *Assessment of a midline episiotomy:* See Box 17-1.
    A. *Position to facilitate assessment:* Ask or assist her in assuming a lateral position with her upper leg flexed on her hip.
    B. *Characteristics to observe:* REEDA: redness, edema, ecchymosis (bruising), drainage, and approximation (intactness); level of hygiene including cleanliness, presence of odor, method used to cleanse perineum and apply the topicals

30. *Recovery room nurse report:* See Table 17-1 for outline of essential information that should be reported regarding the woman, her baby, and the significant

events and findings from her prenatal and childbirth periods.

31. *Signs of potential complications during the postpartum period:* See Signs of Potential Complications Box—Physiologic Problems. Signs are listed according to VS, energy level, uterus, lochia, perineum, legs, breasts, appetite, elimination, rest; note psychosocial complications can also occur (see Chapter 18).

Critical Thinking Exercises

1. *Pain relief for the postpartum woman:* See Comfort subsection of Plan of care and interventions section. Begin by assessing her pain and its characteristics (severity, type, location, relief measures tried and effectiveness) as the basis for action; use a combination of nonpharmacologic and pharmacologic measures; if breastfeeding, administer a systemic analgesic just before or just after breastfeeding.

2. *Woman exhibiting signs of hemorrhage and shock:*
   A. *Criteria to determine if flow was excessive:* See Emergency Box—Hypovolemic Shock and Prevention of bleeding subsection of Plan of care and interventions section. Note length of time the pad was on and the degree to which it is saturated with lochia; check the bed to determine if lochia has pooled there.
   B. *Priority action:* Assess fundus and massage if boggy; once firm, express clots, check bladder for distension and assist to empty, administer oxytocics if ordered
   C. *Nurse's legal responsibility:* Remain with woman and call for help; leaving her in an emergency could lead to a charge of abandonment.
   D. *Additional interventions:* See list of measures in the Emergency Box—Hypovolemic Shock.

3. *Administering rubella vaccine to a post-partum woman:* See Health promotion of future pregnancies and children section. Recheck titer results and order, determine if woman or any household member is immunocompromised, check allergies (duck eggs), inform her of side effects, emphasize that she must not become pregnant for at least three months after the immunization.

4. *Administering RhoGAM to a postpartum woman:* Check woman's and infant's Rh status and results of direct and indirect Coombs test; obtain RhoGAM from blood banks and check all identification data before administration intramuscularly; mother must be Rh negative and infant Rh positive and both Coombs tests must be negative.

5. *Sexual changes after pregnancy and childbirth:* See Sexuality subsection of Discharge teaching section and the Home Care Box—Resumption of Sexual Intercourse. Identify changes that may occur, discuss physical and emotional readiness of the woman, stress importance of open communication, discuss how to prevent discomfort in terms of position and lubrication, and the need to use birth control since the return of ovulation is unpredictable.

6. *Postpartum women:* nursing diagnoses, expected outcomes, and management
   A. *Nursing diagnosis:* risk for infection of episiotomy related to ineffective perineal hygiene measures
   Expected outcome: Episiotomy will heal without infection.
   Management: See Prevention of infection subsection of Plan of care and interventions section and Box 17-3 for full identification of measures to enhance healing and prevent infection.
   B. *Nursing diagnosis:* constipation related to inactivity and lack of knowledge regarding measures to promote elimination during the postpartum period
   Expected outcome: Patient will have bowel movement within two days.
   Management: See Promotion of normal bladder and bowel patterns subsection; determine what she usually does to enhance bowel elimination, encourage activity, roughage, fluids; obtain order for a mild laxative.
   C. *Nursing diagnosis:* pain related to episiotomy and hemorrhoids
   Expected outcome: Patient will experience a reduction in pain following implementation of suggested relief measures.
   Management: See Promotion of comfort subsection and Box 17-3. Emphasize nonpharmacologic relief measures such as perineal care, sitz bath, topicals, side-lying position when in bed, Kegel exercises, measures to enhance bowel and bladder elimination; use pharmacologic measures if local measures are not effective.

7. *Postpartum woman with fundus above umbilicus and off midline*
   A. *Most likely basis:* bladder distention. Confirm by palpating the bladder and asking the woman the last time she voided.
   B. *Nursing action:* Assist woman to empty bladder; measure amount voided and assess characteristics of the urine; palpate bladder and fundus again to determine response; catheterization may be required if she is unable to empty bladder fully, since a distended bladder can lead to hemorrhage and UTIs.

8. *Resumption of physical activity after giving birth:* See Ambulation subsection of Plan of care and interventions section.
   • Assess postanesthesia recovery and physical stability

- Assist and supervise first few times out of bed since orthostatic hypotension can cause her to become dizzy and fall
- Show her where the call light is and what to do if she is alone and begins to feel dizzy or lightheaded

9. *Resumption of full oral intake after giving birth:* See Promotion of nutrition subsection of Plan of care and interventions section. Assess woman for physiologic stability (VS, fundus, lochia, perineum) before resuming full diet; determine type of anesthesia used for birth (if general anesthesia make sure woman is fully alert and gag reflex has returned).

10. *Woman preparing for early discharge*
    A. *Nurse's legal responsibility:* Nurse must assess woman, newborn, and family to confirm that criteria for discharge are fully met. If the criteria are not met the nurse must notify the primary healthcare provider; document all assessment findings, actions, and responses
    B. *Criteria for discharge—maternal, newborn, general:* See Box 17-2.
    C. *Outline essential content that must be taught before discharge:* See Discharge teaching section. Include information regarding self-care, signs of complications, sexual activity, prescribed medications, routine mother and baby check-ups; arrange for a follow-up telephone call and/or a home visit within a day or two of discharge.

11. *Cultural beliefs:* See Impact of cultural diversity subsection in Care management of psychosocial needs section.
    A. *Importance of using a culturally sensitive approach:* Recognition of cultural beliefs and practices is essential to design a plan of care to meet her individual needs; such an approach demonstrates respect, caring, and concern.
    B. *Korean-American woman—heat and cold balance:* Ask woman the sub-

stances and practices she identifies to be hot and cold, then intervene appropriately; see Box 17-4.
    C. *Muslim woman in postpartum period:* See Box 17-4; emphasize diet modification and modesty.

Chapter 18: Adaptation to Parenthood
Chapter Review Activities

1. *Complete table related to maternal adjustment:* Use Table 18-4 and specific subsections for each phase in the Maternal adjustment section.

2. *Complete table related to paternal adjustment:* Use Table 18-5 and Paternal adjustment section.

3. *Attachment of newborn to parents and parents to newborn:* See Parental attachment, bonding, and acquaintance section.
    A. *Define bonding and attachment:*
    Attachment: motivation and commitment of parents and children to decades of supportive and nurturing care of each other
    Bonding: sensitive period after birth when parents have close contact with their infant for optimum development
    B. *Conditions to facilitate attachment:* emotionally healthy parents, competent in communication and caregiving; parent and newborn fit in terms of state, temperament, and gender
    C. *Describe acquaintance process:* Parents use eye contact, touch, talking and exploring to become acquainted; claiming or identification in terms of likeness, differences, and uniqueness is part of this process.

4. *Six parental tasks:* See Parental tasks and responsibilities subsection of Parental role after childbirth section.

5. *Parent-infant contact:* See specific subsection for each form of contact in Parent-Infant contact section.

   Early contact: important to provide time for parents to see, touch, and hold their baby as soon as possible after birth; stress that attachment is an ongoing process. Interference with this early contact because of maternal and/or newborn problems will not have long-term effects.

   Extended contact: Family-centered care, mother-baby care, and use of LDR/LDRP rooms facilitate this type of contact.

6. *Components of the parenting process:* See Parenting process section. Parenting is a process of role attainment and transition that begins with pregnancy and ends when parent is comfortable and confident in the parenting role; nurse should teach, demonstrate, provide time for practice and feedback, arrange for follow-up care, and refer to community agencies and parenting support groups.
   - **Skill/knowledge component:** feeding, holding, clothing, bathing, protecting their newborn are skills that must be learned; parents need a desire to succeed and support from others
   - **Valuing/comfort component:** tenderness, awareness, concern for infant's needs and desires

7. *Periods of parental role attainment during the fourth trimester:* See Parental role after childbirth section.
   - **Early period:** Parents need time to reorganize their lives to include their newborn; focus is on caregiving activities and meeting needs of infant for shelter, nourishment, protection, socialization; characterized by intense learning and need for nurturing.
   - **Consolidation period:** drawing together and uniting of family unit, negotiation of roles, stabilization of tasks, and coming to terms with commitments; becoming in tune with infant

behaviors; competence is growing in care activities

8. claiming, likeness, differences, uniqueness

9. Entrainment, waving of arms, lifting of head, kicking of legs, dancing in tune

10. biorhythmicity, loving care, alert, responsive, social interactions, learning

11. Reciprocity, synchrony

12. rhythm, alert

13. repertoire, gazing, vocalizing, facial expressions, looking, response, infantilize, listen, facial expressions, surprise, happiness, confusion, communicate these emotions

14. responsivity, smiling, cooing, eye contact, en face

15. *Complete table related to parent and infant facilitating and inhibiting behaviors as they relate to attachment:* Use Table 18-1, which covers infant behaviors affecting parent attachment, and Table 18-2, which covers parental behaviors affecting infant attachment.

16. *Factors influencing parents' response to the birth of their child:* Use the information provided in the separate subsections for each of the factors in the Parental responses section.

Critical Thinking Exercises

1. *Teaching parents communication skills with their newborn:* See Communication between parent and infant section.
   A. *Communication techniques:* Discuss touch, eye contact, voice, and odor; demonstrate techniques, have parents try, and point out newborn response in terms of quieting, alerting, making eye contact, gazing; help parents interpret cues.

B. *Baby's communication:* Point out infant responses; discuss processes of entrainment, biorhythmicity, reciprocity, synchrony, and repertoire of behaviors

2. *Woman following emergency cesarean birth; disappointed with lack of immediate bonding time with newborn:*
   - Discuss concepts of early and extended contact
   - Emphasize that the parent-infant attachment process is ongoing—her emotional bond with her baby will not be weaker
   - Help her to meet her own physical and emotional needs so that she develops readiness to meet her newborn's needs
   - Help her to get to know her baby, interact with and care for him or her; point out newborn characteristics including how the baby is responding to her efforts
   - Show her how to communicate with her newborn and how her newborn communicates with her
   - Arrange for follow-up after discharge to see how things are progressing

3. *Sibling adjustment to the newborn:* See Sibling adaptation section and Box 18-4, which identifies strategies parents can use to help their other children adapt; caution her that adjustment takes time and is strongly related to the developmental level and experiences of the sibling(s).

4. *Parents unsure and anxious about caring for their newborn:* Use Table 18-3 and Fig. 18-4. Nursing strategies can include:
   - Performing a newborn assessment with the parents present, pointing out newborn characteristics, and encouraging parents to participate and ask questions
   - Demonstrating newborn care skills and providing time for parents to practice and obtain feedback
   - Providing extended contact with their newborn until discharge
   - Making referrals for follow-up with telephone contacts and home visits; refering to parenting classes and support groups
   - Recommending books, magazines, and videos that discuss newborns

5. *Parental disappointment with newborn's gender and/or appearance:* See Parental tasks and responsibilities section. Foster attachment and claiming; help parents to get acquainted with the infant and to reconcile the real child with the fantasy child; discuss the basis for the molding, caput, and forceps marks and how they will be resolved; be alert for problems with attachment and care so follow-up can be arranged.

6. *Grandparent adjustment:* see Grandparent adaptation section. Observe interaction between grandparents and parents taking note of signs of effective interaction and conflict; involve grandparents in teaching sessions as appropriate; spend time with grandparents to help them to be supportive without "taking over" or being critical; help the new parents to recognize the unique role grandparents can play as parenting role models, nurturers, and providers of respite care.

7. *Woman experiencing postpartum blues:*
   - *Nursing diagnosis:* ineffective coping, related to hormonal changes and increased responsibilities
   - *Expected outcome:* Woman will report feeling more content with her new role following use of recommended coping strategies.
   - *Nursing management:* See Home Care Box—Coping with postpartum blues. Involve both Jane and her husband in the teaching and development of a plan for coping with the blues; this must occur early to prevent development of postpartum depression.

Chapter 19: Immediate Care of the Newborn

Chapter Review Activities

1. P

2. N

3. N

4. P

5. N

6. N

7. N

8. N

9. P

10. N

11. N

12. N

13. P

14. N

15. N

16. N

17. P

18. N

19. N

20. N

21. P

22. N

23. N

24. *Newborn's establishment of respirations*
   A. *Factors initiating breathing after birth:* reflex triggered by such factors as pressure changes, chilling, noise, light, and other sensations associated with exposure to extrauterine life; chemoreceptor activation by lowered oxygen level, higher carbon dioxide level, and lower pH
   B. *Conditions essential for maintaining an adequate oxygen supply:* removal of lung fluid, synchronous expansion of chest and abdomen, patent airway, and sufficient surfactant
   C. *Expected newborn respiratory pattern:* shallow, irregular rate of 30 to 60 breaths per minute, short periods of apnea less than 15 seconds, loud and clear breath sounds
   D. *Signs of respiratory distress:* See Signs of Potential Complications Box—Abnormal Breathing. Signs include nasal flaring, retractions and increased use of intercostal muscles, grunting with expiration, seesaw respirations, rate of less than 30 or more than 60 breaths per minute at rest, apnea of more than 15 seconds, adventitious breath sounds
   E. *Three methods of relieving airway obstruction:* See Emergency Box—Relieving Airway Obstruction. Methods: back blows, turning infant, chest thrusts

25. *Complete table related to closure of fetal circulatory shunts:* See Circulatory system subsection of Physiologic adjustments for method of closure and Fig. 8-8 for location and purpose.

26. *Newborn—cold stress:* See Effects of cold stress subsection of Thermoregulation section and Fig. 19-2.
   A. *Dangers of cold stress:* metabolic and physiologic demands on the newborn increase → increased oxygen need/con-

sumption → oxygen and energy are diverted from brain cell and cardiac function and growth → decreased oxygen leads to vasoconstriction, respiratory distress and reopening of the ductus arteriosus → acidosis and increased level of bilirubin

B. *Newborn behaviors associated with cold stress:* increased respiratory rate, cyanosis, decrease in oxygen, pH and glucose levels, signs of acidosis

C. *Measures to stabilize newborn temperature:* See Maintenance of body temperature subsection of Plan of care and interventions; implement measures that reflect application of health loss mechanisms.
   - Dry infant and cover with warmed blankets or wrap with mother on her abdomen
   - Cover head
   - Use radiant heat shield/warmer to stabilize temperature, assess newborn and perform procedures
   - Adjust environment

D. *Guidelines for using a radiant heat shield:* See Maintenance of body temperature subsection of Care management from birth through the first 2 hours section; answer should include placing the unclothed newborn under the warmer, correctly attaching the probe and setting the warmer, and monitoring the axillary temperature periodically.

27. *Heat loss mechanisms—definitions and nursing measures:* see Table 19-2 and Heat loss subsection of Thermoregulation section.

28. Characteristics of physiologic jaundice; See Physiologic jaundice subsection of Hepatic system section for a listing of the most common characteristics; major characteristic is the appearance of jaundice after the first 24 hours of life.

29. sleep, wake, deep, light, drowsy, quiet alert, active alert, crying, quiet alert, smiling, vocalizing, moving in synchrony with speech, watching parents' faces, responding to voices, internal, external, responses, organize behavior

30. *Complete table related to phases of a newborn's transition to extrauterine life:* See Transition period subsection of Behavioral adaptations section for identification of each phase and description of timing/duration and typical newborn behaviors for each phase.

31. *Two measures to prevent or limit physiologic hyperbilirubinemia:* See Physiologic jaundice subsection of Hepatic system section.
   - Early feeding: stimulates gastrocolic reflex, leading to passage of meconium, which contains bilirubin that would otherwise be absorbed into the circulatory system
   - Prevent cold stress since acidosis frees bilirubin

32. *Nurse's responsibility in identification of newborn after birth:* See Identification subsection of Immediate interventions section. Complete the identification process before mother and newborn are separated; apply matching ID bands to both immediately after birth; newborn's footprint and mother's fingerprints go on a footprint form.

33. T

34. F

35. T

36. F

37. T

38. T

39. T

40. F

41. F

42. F

43. F

44. T

45. T

46. T

47. F

48. F

49. T

50. F

51. F

Crossword puzzle

Across: 1. Suck; 2. Habituation; 5. RBC; 7. Suture; 9. Milia; 11. Extrusion; 12. Rugae; 13. One; 14. Colic; 16. Brick; 19. Jaundice; 22. Mongolian spots; 23. Harlequin; 25. Gluteal; 28. Two; 29. Vernix caseosa; 30. LGA; 31. SGA; 33. Tonic neck; 34. Tremor; 38. Grasp; 39. Ovale; 40. Smegma; 43. Brown fat; 45. Surfactant; 46. Convection; 49. Evaporation; 50. Peeling; 51. Reflexes

Down: 1. Strabismus; 3. Three; 4. Moro; 6. Flare; 8. Murmur; 9. Meconium; 10. Acrocyanosis; 15. Lanugo; 17. Hydrocele; 18. Telangiectatic; 20. Cephalhematoma; 21. Pearl; 24. Babinski; 26. Molding; 27. Petechiae; 32. Rooting; 35. AGA; 36. Apgar; 37. Reactivity; 41. Conduction; 42. Gastrocolic; 44. Toxicum; 47. Creases; 48. Pad

Critical Thinking Exercises

1. *Apgar scoring*

   Baby boy Smith: Heart rate: 120 (2); respiratory effort: good (2); muscle tone: active movement (2); reflex: irritability cry with stimulus (2); color: acrocyanosis (1). Score: 9. Interpretation: score of 7 to 10 indicates that infant will have no difficulty adjusting to extrauterine life.

   Baby girl Doe: Heart rate: 102 (2); respiratory effort: slow, irregular (1); muscle tone: some flexion (1); reflex: irritability grimace response to stimulus (1); color: pale (0). Score: 5. Interpretation: score of 4 to 6 indicates moderate difficulty adjusting to extrauterine life.

2. *Complete table related to physiologic functioning of newborn compared to that of an adult:* Use specific subsection for each function in the Physiologic adjustment section.

3. *Parental concern regarding head variations:* See Caput succedaneum and Cephalhematoma subsections of Integumentary system and Molding in skeletal system sections. Discuss each finding in terms of cause, significance for the newborn's health status and adjustment, and how/when it will be resolved. Refer to Figs. 19-4 and 19-8 to facilitate the parents' understanding.

4. *Parental concern regarding "bruises" on newborn's back and buttocks:* Discuss the characteristics and cause of mongolian spots. See Mongolian spots subsection of Integumentary system section.

5. *Newborn with mucus in airway:* See Maintaining a patent airway subsection of Stabilization and resuscitation section.
   A. *Nursing diagnosis:* impaired gas exchange related to upper airway obstruction with mucus
   B. *Steps for using bulb syringe:* Suction mouth first, then nose, and compress bulb before insertions. Insert tip along side of mouth (not over tongue), which could stimulate the gag reflex; continue until breathing sounds clear. Teach parents how to use a bulb syringe.

C. *Guidelines for use of mechanical suction:* Suction for 10 seconds or less per insertion, use 80 mm Hg setting, and lubricate catheter with sterile water. Insert along base of tongue or horizontally through nose into nares; repeat until breathing sounds clear.

6. *Assessment of newborn girl*
   A. *Protocol for assessment during first two hours:* Use Table 19-3 (Apgar score), Box 19-1 (Initial Physical Assessment by Body System), and Initial Assessment and nursing diagnoses section.
   B. *Two priority nursing diagnoses:* Consider nursing diagnoses related to ineffective airway clearance, airway obstruction, hypothermia, ineffective thermoregulation.
   C. *Priority nursing care measures:* Discuss each of these areas.
      - Stabilization of respiration and airway patency
      - Maintenance of body temperature
      - Immediate interventions in terms of identification, prophylactic medications, promotion of bonding

7. *Maternal concern regarding breastfeeding and jaundice:* See Physiologic jaundice and Jaundice associated with breastfeeding subsection in Hepatic system section.
   - Explain cause and reassure mother that it is a physiologic condition that does not have a negative impact on the newborn
   - Tell her when it might occur and when it will disappear
   - Discuss what can be done to prevent or limit its occurrence: feed the newborn eight times per day around the clock since colostrum is a natural laxative that promotes expulsion of bilirubin containing meconium

Chapter 20: Assessment and Care of the Newborn
Chapter Review Activities

1. F
2. T
3. F
4. T
5. F
6. T
7. F
8. T
9. F
10. T
11. F
12. T
13. F
14. T
15. T
16. F
17. T
18. F
19. T
20. F
21. Ortolani's maneuver
22. Vitamin K, 0.5-1 mg, 25, 5/8

23. prepuce (foreskin), phimosis, foreskin, glans penis, urinary tract infection, penile cancer, parents

24. Habituation, environmental stimuli, constant, repetitive, decreased

25. Orientation

26. Range of state, regulation of state

27. Motor performance

28. Autonomic stability

29. Consolability, hand to mouth movements, alerting, voices, noises, visual

30. Cuddliness

31. inborn errors of metabolism, phenylketonuria (PKU), milk, 24 hours, galactosemia, glucose, failure to thrive, mental retardation, cataracts, jaundice, hepatomegaly, cirrhosis of the liver, hypothyroidism

32. *Assessment of gestational age:* See Assessment of clinical gestational age section and Figs. 20-1 and 20-2.
   A. *List signs of neuromuscular maturity:* Assess such signs as posture, arm recoil, popliteal angle, scarf sign, heel to ear. Use column no. 4 for full-term newborn; note that the full-term newborn is more flexed and resists efforts to pull limbs in a certain direction (e.g., bringing the newborn's heel to his or her ear or his or her elbow across the sternum).
   B. *Signs of physical maturity:* Assess such signs as skin condition, presence of lanugo, plantar creases, breast size, eye and ear formation, condition of genitalia. Use column no. 4 for expected findings for a full-term newborn.
   C. 12, 96
   D. *Designation of AGA, LGA, SGA:* See Weight related to gestational subsec-

tion of Assessment and nursing diagnoses section.
   • First: determine gestational age using the new Ballard Scale (Fig. 20-1A)
   • Second: measure newborn's head circumference, length, and weight
   • Third: plot estimated gestational age and measurements on graph (Fig. 20-1B) to determine classification

33. *Health teaching in preparation for discharge:* See Home Care Box—Sponge Bathing and specific subsection for each topic in Discharge planning and teaching—anticipatory guidance section.

34. *Safety and medical aseptic principles when sponge-bathing newborn:* Use Home Care Box—Sponge Bathing.
   Medical asepsis: Wash head to toe, inner to outer canthus, genitalia from front to back. Avoid soap (especially harsh soap), change diapers promptly, care for cord and circumcision site.
   Safety: Prevent heat loss, gather all supplies before starting, never leave infant alone, never hold newborn under running water.

35. *Factors influencing newborn behavior:* See appropriate subsection in Behavioral characteristics—other factors influencing behavior of newborns section for a description of how gestational age, time, stimuli, medication, ethnicity, and sensory behaviors influence newborn's behavior.

36. *Complete table regarding newborn reflexes:* Use Table 20-2, which describes each reflex in terms of stimulus required and expected response.

37. *Guidelines for weighing and measuring infant:* Use Table 21-1, Figs. 20-3 and 20-5, and Baseline measurements subsection of physical examination section. Wear gloves if performed before first bath.

Weight: balance scale, cover with scale paper, place undressed infant on scale, keep hand hovering over infant, never turn away

Head circumference: use disposable paper tape, measure at widest part of head just above ears and eyebrow; repeat if molding is present at birth

Chest circumference: use disposable paper tape, measure across nipple line

Abdominal circumference: use disposable paper tape, measure at level of umbilicus

Length: use disposable paper tape, measure from crown to rump, then rump to heels

38. Brazelton Neonatal Behavioral Assessment Scale (BNBAS) and Mother's Assessment of the Behavior of her Infant (MABI): See Assessment of infant behavior section.
    A. *Purpose of using these scales*:
       - Initial and ongoing systematic method of assessment of newborn behavior; interactive examination to determine infant's neurologic and behavioral responses to 28 areas organized into clusters
       - Assess initial parent-infant relationship
       - Guide for parents to help them focus on their infant's individuality, develop a deeper attachment and more positive perception, and increase infant-parent interaction
    B. *Clusters of neonatal behaviors assessed with the BNBAS:* See Box 20-1.

39. *Creation of a protective environment in terms of infection control and safety:* See Protective environment subsection of Plan of care and interventions.
    Environment: adequate lighting, ventilation, warmth, and humidity; elimination of fire hazards, safety with electrical appliances
    Infection control: use standard precautions correctly, adequate floor space to keep bassinets 60 cm apart, separate areas for cleaning and storing equipment and supplies, keep persons with infection away or use appropriate precautions
    Safety: security measures, identification measures, instruction of parents

Critical Thinking Exercises

1. *Performing a physical examination of newborn before discharge*
   A. *Information required from maternal health history and prenatal and intrapartal records:* See Maternal record review subsection of Physical assessment section and Fig. 20-2.
   B. *Actions to ensure safety and accuracy:* well-lighted, warm and draft-free environment, undress as needed, place on firm, flat surface with constant supervision, place under warmer if needed, progress in a systematic manner from cleanest to dirtiest area
   C. *Major areas assessed:* See Tables 20-1 and 20-2. Areas include general appearance, VS, baseline measurements, integument, abdomen, back, genitalia, anus, extremities, neurologic, behavioral characteristics.
   D. *Rationale for presence of parents:* chance to observe parent-infant interactions, identify and meet learning needs, foster active involvement in assessment and care of their infant, encourage discussion of questions and concerns, chance to explain newborn characteristics and capabilities

2. *Care of circumcision site and cord*
   A. *Nursing diagnosis:* risk for infection related to removal of foreskin and healing of umbilical cord site
   B. *Expected outcome:* Cord and circumcision sites will heal without infection.
   C. *Teaching about care:* See Home Care Box—Circumcision and Home Care Box and Sponge bathing cord care section. Emphasize importance of assessing sites for progress of healing and

signs of infection; discuss measures to keep the area clean and dry and to enhance comfort; teach parents how to assess circumcision site for bleeding and what to do if it occurs, and how to assess urination and what to do if newborn has difficulty voiding.

3. *Parental concern about newborn weight loss:* Determine percentage of weight loss, making sure it does not exceed 10%. Explain that their newborn's weight loss of 6% is well within the expected range; discuss the cause of the loss and feeding measures, and inform them that the birth weight will be regained within two weeks

4. *Newborn with hyperbilirubinemia:* See Therapy for hyperbilirubinemia section and Teaching Guidelines Box—Hyperbilirubinemia.
   A. *Respond to parent's concern:* Tell parents in simple terms that their newborn is exhibiting physiologic jaundice, and explain its cause and its common occurrence.
   B. *Identify expected findings of physiologic hyperbilirubinemia:* jaundice; watery, greenish stool; and sleepiness. See Chapter 19.
   C. *Precautions and care measures during phototherapy:* Increase fluids, feed at least every 3 hr, cover eyes (remove covering periodically to check eyes), monitor temperature, cleanse stools promptly (do not use lotions), place uncovered under lights and change position periodically, and remove from lights for feeding, cuddling, and eye contact.

5. *Parental interest in newborn's sensory capabilities:* See Sensory behaviors subsection of Behavioral characteristics—other factors influencing behavior of newborns section.
   A. *What nurse should tell parents:* Discuss newborn's capability regarding vision, hearing, touch, taste, and smell.

   B. *Stimuli parents can provide to facilitate their newborn's development:* face to face/eye contact, objects (especially those that are bright or have black and white patterns), talking to infant, music, heartbeat simulator, touch, infant massage

6. *Assessment of the progress in parent-infant attachment*
   A. *Attachment behaviors to observe:* See Teaching Guidelines Box—Assessing attachment behaviors; many behaviors described could form a quick assessment tool.
   B. *Factors influencing development of attachment:*
      • Expectations about infant (fantasy vs. real child)
      • Manner in which parents were parented
      • Planned versus unplanned or unwanted pregnancy
      • Perception of the effect the infant will have on their lives
      • Reaction to newborn; availability of support system
      • Events of pregnancy and childbirth; condition of the mother
      • Progress of breastfeeding
      • Availability of opportunities for close contact with newborn including rooming in, mother-baby care, liberal visiting hours for family members

Chapter 21: Newborn Nutrition and Feeding

Chapter Review Activities

1. *Calculate energy and fluid requirements of three newborns:* Use the following formulas:
   • 108 Kcal/kg/day first six months of life
   • 98 Kcal/kg/day second six months of life
   • 150 ml/kg/day fluid

Jim (1 month, 4 kg): 432 Kcal/day; 600 ml of fluid
Sue (4 months, 6 kg): 648 Kcal/day; 900 ml of fluid
Sam (7 months, 7.5 kg): 735 Kcal/day; 1,125 ml of fluid

2. *Label illustration of lactation structures:* See Fig. 21-1. A, alveolus; B, ductule; C, duct; D, lactiferous duct; E, lactiferous sinus; F, nipple pore; G, ampulla; H, areola

3. *Identification of advantages of breastfeeding:* See Benefits of breastfeeding section.

4. *Describe four breastfeeding positions:* See Home Care Box—Breastfeeding and Positioning subsection of Plan of care and interventions. Describe football hold, cradle and modified cradle or across the lap position, and the side-lying position.

5. *Feeding readiness cues:* See Feeding readiness section.
   A. *Cues:* hand-to-mouth or hand-to-hand movements, sucking motions, strong rooting reflex, mouthing
   B. *Rationale for feeding according to these cues:* If cues are missed baby may cry vigorously, become distraught, or withdraw into sleep; these behaviors will make feeding more difficult or impossible.

6. *Differences between foremilk and hindmilk:* See Uniqueness of human milk section. **Foremilk:** bluish-white, part skim and part whole-milk lactose, protein, water-soluble vitamins; **hindmilk:** cream is "let down" into the feeding, denser in calories from fat to ensure optimal growth and contentment between feedings

7. *Label illustrations of reflexes:*
   Milk production reflex: A, sucking stimulus; B, hypothalamus; C, anterior pituitary gland (prolactin); D, milk production
   Let-down reflex: A, sucking stimulus;

B, hypothalamus; C, posterior pituitary gland (oxytocin); D, let-down reflex

8. *Stages of lactogenesis:* See Uniqueness of human milk section.
   Stage I: Begins in pregnancy when breasts are prepared for milk production and colostrum is formed in the breasts
   Stage II: Colostrum changes to mature milk; "milk coming in" on the third to fifth day after birth; onset of copious milk production
   Stage III: Milk changes over about 10 days when the mature milk is established

9. *AWHONN Guidelines for Breastfeeding:* Box 21-1 lists the recommended guidelines.

10. *Proper latch on:* See Latching on subsection of Plan of care and interventions—breastfeeding section.
    A. *Steps to ensure proper latch on:* hold baby close to breast, tickle baby's lower lip to simulate rooting reflex, tongue extrudes, pull baby onto nipple and areola
    B. *Signs of proper latch on:* firm, tugging sensation on nipple, no pinching or pain, baby's cheeks are rounded, jaw glides smoothly with sucking

11. F

12. F

13. T

14. T

15. F

16. T

17. F

18. T

19. T

20. T

21. F

22. T

23. F

24. T

25. T

26. T

27. F

28. F

29. *Calming a fussy baby:* See Bottles and pacifiers subsection of Special consideration section.

30. *Complete table related to assessment of infant and mother regarding breastfeeding:* Use Infant and mother assessment and nursing diagnoses section.

Crossword puzzle

Across: 1, mastitis; 3, massage; 8, lactogenesis; 10, confusion; 11, milk glands; 12, lactation consultant; 15, demand; 16, engorgement; 17, feeding readiness cues; 19, weaning; 22, everted; 25, colostrum; 27, milk duct; 28, prolactin

Down: 2, shell; 4, shut down; 5, growth spurt; 6, monilial; 7, football; 9, areola; 12, lactiferous sinuses; 13, cradle; 14, let down; 18, inverted; 20, alveoli; 21, oxytocin; 23, rooting; 24, extrusion; 26, latch on

Critical Thinking Exercises

1. *Analysis of breastfeeding technique:* (+) *indicates competency;* (−) *indicates need for further instruction.*
   A. −
   B. +
   C. −
   D. −
   E. +
   F. −
   G. +
   H. +
   I. −
   J. −
   K. +
   L. −

2. *Bottle-feeding mother wishes to give her newborn skim milk to prevent cardiac problems:* See Fat subsection of Nutrient needs section. Emphasize the importance of fat in the newborn's diet for energy and supplying essential fatty acids for growth and tissue maintenance, cell membranes, and hormone production. At least 15% of calories must come from fat; skim milk lacks essential fatty acids.

3. *Infant feeding method decision-making during prenatal period:* See Choosing an infant feeding method section.
   A. *Rationale for couple making the decision together:* Both should learn about the pros and cons of feeding methods with an emphasis on the benefits of breastfeeding and how the partner can help with the method.
   B. *Making the decision prenatally:* The prenatal period is a less stressful time, allowing for full consideration of options, how feeding methods would be incorporated into life activities (such as work outside the home), and learning about breastfeeding by attending classes and reading.
   C. *How nurse can facilitate the decision-making process:* Provide information about feeding methods in a nonjudgmental manner, dispel myths, address personal concerns of the couple, and make needed referrals to WIC, lactation consultant, breastfeeding classes, and the La Leche League.

4. *Breastfeeding mother's questions and concerns:* See Milk production subsection of

Overview of lactation section (A, B), Teaching Guidelines Box—Common Breastfeeding Problems (D, E).

A. *Breast size:* Discuss development of lactation structures during pregnancy; emphasize the importance of this development, not the size of the breasts.

B. *Let-down reflex:* Explain what it is and why it happens (including physical and emotional triggers), and why it is so important in terms of the hindmilk that the baby receives.

C. *Signs that breastfeeding is going well:* See Box 21-2, which identifies maternal and fetal indicators of effective breastfeeding during the first week following birth, and Box 21-3, which lists signs of adequate intake by the newborn.

D. *Nipple soreness:* Discuss and demonstrate measures to prevent and treat sore nipples including, most importantly, good breastfeeding techniques such as latch on, removal, and alternating breasts and positions, and breast care measures such as air-drying nipples, avoiding soap, and applying colostrum then breast milk after feeding.

E. *Engorgement:* Prevention measures include frequency of feeding every 2 to 3 hours with 15 to 20 minutes on each breast. Treatment measures include warm packs and massage before feeding, ice afterwards, cabbage leaves, and support.

F. *Afterpains and increased flow:* Explain that oxytocin is released as a result of newborn sucking. This hormone triggers the let down reflex but also stimulates the uterus to contract, causing afterpains in the first three to five days after birth. Oxytocin also reduces excessive bleeding.

G. *Breastfeeding as a birth control method:* See Effect of menstruation and Breastfeeding and contraception subsections of Care of mother section.

Emphasize that breastfeeding is not an effective contraceptive method: although ovulation may be delayed, its return is unpredictable and may occur before the first menstrual period. Discuss contraceptive methods that are safe to use with breastfeeding.

H. *Weaning:* See Weaning section. Emphasize that weaning needs to be a gradual process, eliminating one feeding at a time.

5. *Starting solid foods:* See Introduction of solid food section. Emphasize importance of waiting to introduce solids at four to six months of age, when the infant is developmentally ready; early introduction of solid foods can lead to allergies, excessive caloric intake, and diminished interest in breastfeeding. Dispel myth that solids encourage sleeping through the night.

6. *Infrequent feeding of sleeping baby:* See Frequency and duration of feeding and Special considerations subsections of Plan of care and interventions—breastfeeding section. Discuss feeding readiness cues to facilitate proper timing of feedings (which should occur every three hours during the day and every four hours at night for a total of eight to 10 feedings per day); discuss techniques to wake sleeping baby.

7. *Bottle-feeding mother:* See Formula feeding section and Home Care Box—Formula Preparation and Feeding.

A. *Nurse's response to mother's concern:* Discuss how the mother can facilitate close contact and socializing with the infant during feeding: sit comfortably, touch, talk, sing, and read to the infant to make feeding an intimate and pleasant experience for both.

B. *Guidelines for bottle-feeding:* Include instruction related to amount and frequency; how to prepare formula and bottles/nipples; and principles of feeding including the semi-upright position, not propping bottles, fluid filling the nipple, cues of satiety, burping, and choosing a formula type.

Chapter 22: Assessment for Risk Factors

Chapter Review Activities

1. F

2. T

3. T

4. T

5. F

6. F

7. T

8. F

9. T

10. T

11. F

12. T

13. T

14. F

15. T

16. F

17. T

18. F

19. *Factors placing a pregnant woman and her fetus/newborn at risk:* Box 22-1 describes several risk factors in each category: biophysical, psychosocial, sociodemographic, and environmental.

20. *Regionalization of health care:* See Regionalization of health care Services section.
    A. *Advantages:* Cost-effective approach can result in more favorable maternal and fetal/newborn outcomes since each hospital cannot provide the full spectrum of services required in both low-risk and high-risk pregnancies.
    B. *Purposes and goals of each level:*
       Level I facilities: manage low-risk pregnancy and childbirth; early identification of high-risk pregnancy and newborn; provide stabilization care in obstetric and neonatal emergencies
       Level II facilities: care for specified types of maternal and neonatal complications; full range of uncomplicated maternity and neonatal care
       Level III facilities: capacity to manage complex maternal and neonatal disorders; women are often transported before birth to optimize maternal and fetal/neonatal outcome; outreach education for health care providers

21. *Nonstress test (NST) and Contraction stress test (CST):* See Electronic fetal monitoring section.
    A. *State rationale for performing these tests in the third trimester:* Goal is to determine if the intrauterine environment is supportive of the fetus and for the timing of childbirth, especially if the risk for uteroplacental insufficiency is present. Fetal neurologic system is capable of producing the expected result (e.g., accelerations with fetal movement [NST] and fetus is of a gestational age when birth can be accomplished with a fairly good outcome).
    B. *Indications for tests:* Many reasons are listed in the Indications subsection, including preexisting and pregnancy-induced maternal health problems that could interfere with uteroplacental circulation.

C. *Contraindications for CST:* ROM, previous classic cesarean incision, history of preterm labor/birth, placenta previa, abruptio placenta.

22. *Nurse's role in ultrasound examination:* See Ultrasonography section. Instruct woman to come with full bladder, explain purpose and method of examination, and assist her into a supine position with shoulder elevated and hip slightly tilted. Watch for supine hypotension when lying down and orthostatic hypotension when rising, indicate how the fetus is being measured, and point out fetus and its movements.

23. *State one risk factor for each pregnancy problem listed:* See Box 22-3, which lists several risk factors for each category including preterm labor, polyhydramnios, IUGR, postterm pregnancy, and chromosomal abnormalities.

24. C

25. E

26. A

27. H

28. I

29. B

30. D

31. J

32. F

33. G

34. K

Crossword puzzle

Across: 2, amniocentesis; 4, biparietal; 6, nonstress; 8, alphafetoprotein; 11, ultrasonography; 13, nonreactive; 14, negative; 16, phosphatidyl-glycerol; 17, Coombs; 18, fetal movements; 19, alarm signal; 20, chorionic villus
Down: 1, contractions stress; 3, nipple; 4, biophysical profile; 5, positive; 7, reactive; 9, APT; 10, RhoGAM; 12, LS; 15, triple marker

Critical Thinking Exercises

1. Woman having a Biophysical Profile performed: See Table 22-3 for identification of the variables assessed and how the test is scored.
   A. *Nurse's response to woman's concern about the test:* Describe how the test will be performed using ultrasonography and external electronic monitoring. Explain that the purpose is to view the fetus within its environment and to determine how it moves and how its heart rate responds to activity.
   B. *Meaning of a score of 8:* A score of 8 to 10 is a normal result.

2. *Amniocentesis:* See Amniocentesis section and Nurse's role in antepartal assessment for risk section.
   A. *Preparing woman:* Explain procedure, witness an informed consent, assess maternal vital signs and general health status, FHR prior to the test. Ensure that ultrasound is performed to locate placenta and fetus prior to the test.
   B. *Supporting woman during the procedure:* Explain what is happening and what she will feel, help her to relax, and assess her reactions.
   C. *Postprocedure care and instructions:* Monitor maternal VS and status, FHR, and when test results will be ready and whom to call; provide RhoGAM since the mother is Rh negative and her husband is Rh positive; teach her to check for signs of infection, bleeding, rupture of membranes, and contractions; make a follow-up phone call.

3. *Nonstress test:* See Nonstress test subsection of Electronic fetal monitoring section.

A. *Preparation:* Explain what the test is, what will happen, and why it is performed. Choose time when fetus is usually awake.

B. *Indicate how the test is conducted:* Place in seated or semi-Fowler's position, observe for and prevent supine hypotension, attach external fetal monitor, instruct mother to indicate fetal movement, assess change, if any, in FHR as a result of movement.

C. *Analyze results:* See Table 22-5 for criteria used to determine test results and Fig. 22-8 for a monitor tracing.

  (1) Indicates a reactive result: good variability with normal baseline range and accelerations as defined

  (2) Indicates a nonreactive result: no accelerations with limited variability

4. *Contraction stress test:* See Contraction stress test subsection of Electronic fetal monitoring section.

A. *Preparation:* Assess woman's vital signs, general health status, and contraindications for the test; attach external monitor and assess FHR and uterine activity; explain purpose of test and what it entails; assist her into position as for NST.

B. *Indicate how the test is performed:* See Protocol for a Nipple Stimulation Contraction Stress Test. Three UC must occur within a 10 minute period; make sure that contractions subside after the test and assess maternal and fetal responses.

C. *Indicate how oxytocin contraction stress test would be performed:* See Protocol for Oxytocin Stimulated Contraction Stress test.

D. *Analysis of results:* See Table 22-6 for criteria used to interpret test results.

  (1) Negative result (see Fig. 22-9*A*): no late deceleration patterns noted

  (2) Positive result (see Fig. 22-9*B*): late decelerations with the appropriate number of contractions, limited variability

Chapter 23: Pregnancy at Risk: Preexisting Conditions

Chapter Review Activities

1. *Physiologic basis for clinical manifestations of diabetes mellitus:* See Diabetes mellitus—pathogenesis section for a full explanation of hyperglycemia, polyuria, glycosuria, polydipsia, weight loss, and polyphagia in terms of cause and how they interrelate.

2. hyperglycemia, insulin secretion, insulin action, both

3. Polyuria, polydipsia, polyphagia, glycosuria

4. Pregestational diabetes mellitus, gestational diabetes

5. glucose control, euglycemia (normoglycemia)

6. hypoglycemia, hypoglycemic, nausea, vomiting, cravings, glucose

7. hyperglycemia, ketoacidosis, insulin, 14 to 16 weeks

8. phosphatidylglycerol, lecithin, sphingomyelin

9. glycosylated hemoglobin

10. blood glucose, 30 to 35, 50 to 60 percent, simple, complex, 12 to 20 percent, 20 to 30 percent

11. breakfast, lunch, dinner, bedtime, postprandial, second, third, increased

12. $\frac{2}{3}$, before breakfast, NPH, regular, $\frac{1}{3}$, before dinner, hypoglycemia, short acting, before dinner, longer acting, bedtime

13. *Maternal risks/complications and fetal and neonatal risks/complications related to pregestational diabetes:* See Maternal risks/

complications subsection and Fetal and newborn risks/complications subsection.

Maternal: increased rate of childbirth complications, PIH, hydramnios, postpartum hemorrhage, infection, hypoglycemia and ketoacidosis

Fetal/newborn: congenital anomalies, macrosomia with related birth injuries, IUGR, RDS, neonatal hypoglycemia, hypocalcemia, hyperbilirubinemia

14. *Complete table related to metabolic changes of pregnancy and impact of these changes on pregnancy:* See Metabolic changes associated with pregnancy subsection of Diabetes mellitus section for full description related to each stage of pregnancy including the antepartal trimesters and the postpartum period.

15. *State effect of thyroid disorders on reproduction and pregnancy:* See Thyroid disorders section for a full description of hyperthyroidism and hypothyroidism; consider effects of these disorders on reproductive development, sexuality, fertility in terms of ability to conceive and to sustain a pregnancy, potential fetal/newborn complications related to maternal treatment of her thyroid disorder.

16. T

17. F

18. T

19. T

20. F

21. F

22. F

23. T

24. T

25. T

26. F

27. F

28. F

29. F

30. F

31. F

Crossword puzzle

Across: 1, glucose tolerance; 5, cerclage; 6, hyperreflexia; 9, preeclampsia; 11, ectopic; 14, normoglycemia; 15, venospasm; 16, HELLP; 17, intrauterine growth; 18, subinvolution; 21, glycosylated; 24, gestational; 25, molar; 27, hematoma; 28, macrosomia; 29, ketoacidosis

Down: 2, edema; 3, eclampsia; 4, protein; 6, hypoglycemia; 7, pregestational; 8, atony; 10, clonus; 12, incompetent; 13, previa; 19, insulin; 20, hyperemesis; 22, abortion; 23, hydramnios; 26, abruptio

32. T

33. F

34. T

35. T

36. T

37. F

38. F

39. T

40. F

41. T

42. T

43. T

44. F

45. T

46. F

47. F

48. T

49. F

50. F

51. T

52. T

53. T

54. T

55. F

56. *Maternal and fetal complications related to maternal cardiovascular disease:* See Cardiovascular disorders section. Complications can include increase in spontaneous abortion, incidence of preterm labor and birth, IUGR, maternal mortality, and stillbirth.

57. *Factors placing woman at high risk for HIV infection:* See HIV and AIDS section. Factors include IV drug use and heterosexual contact with a high-risk man.

58. *Factors that increase risk of perinatal HIV transmission:* See Box 23-2.

59. F

60. T

61. T

62. F

63. T

64. F

65. T

Critical Thinking Exercises

1. *Preconception counseling for a diabetic woman:* See Preconception counseling subsection in Diabetes mellitus section.
   - Discuss purpose in terms of planning the optimum time for her pregnancy (when she has established glucose control within normal limits, since this will significantly decrease the incidence of congenital anomalies); diagnose any vascular problems; emphasize importance of her health and well-being prior to pregnancy for a healthy outcome
   - Discuss how her diabetic management will need to be altered during pregnancy; include her husband since his health is important, as is his support of her during pregnancy

2. *Pregnant woman with pregestational diabetes experiencing hypoglycemia:* see Table 23-1, Home Care Box—Treatment for Hypoglycemia, and Metabolic changes associated with pregnancy and Pregestational diabetes mellitus subsections of the Diabetes mellitus section.
   A. *Problem*: Signs and symptoms suggest hypoglycemia resulting from insufficient caloric intake with no adjustment in insulin dosage.
   B. *Action:* Check blood glucose level if possible, eat or drink something that contains a simple carbohydrate, rest for 15 minutes and recheck blood glucose, repeat if glucose remains low.

3. *Woman with pregestational diabetes:* care management
   A. *Additional fetal assessment measures:* See Fetal surveillance subsection for a discussion of a variety of antepartal tests for fetus. Tests can include ultrasound examinations, maternal serum AFP, fetal echocardiography, Doppler blood flow analysis through cord, maternal daily fetal movement counts, NST, BPP, and CST.

B. *Stressors facing woman and her family:* alteration in daily living including usual diabetes management, need for additional antepartal testing and prenatal visits, financial implications

C. *Complete table related to care management during antepartum, intrapartum and postpartum periods:* See specific subsections for diet, glucose monitoring, and insulin in the Plan of care and intervention—Diabetes mellitus section. Use Home Care Boxes in this section for additional suggestions for nursing interventions including health teaching; Plan of care for a woman with diabetes may also be helpful.

D. *Activity/exercise recommendations:* See Exercise subsection of Plan of care and interventions—Diabetes mellitus section. Recommend exercise according to her diabetic status; discuss when she should exercise and emphasize the importance of checking her blood glucose level before, during, and after and adjusting calorie intake and insulin administration accordingly.

E. *Birth control recommendations:* See Postpartum subsection. Discuss risks and benefits of methods including their impact on glucose levels (hormone-based) and infection (barrier methods such as diaphragm and cervical cap). Barrier method is preferred, starting with condom and spermicide until diaphragm can be fitted; stress importance of waiting until healing is complete to prevent infection.

4. *Hispanic woman with gestational diabetes:* See Gestational diabetes section.

A. *Complication with validating findings:* gestational diabetes; 50 gm glucose test result 152 mg/dl (≥ 140 mg/dl). Glucose tolerance test results reveal three values exceeding the normal range (fasting, one hour result, three hour result). See Fig 23-4.

B. *List risk factors:* over 30 years of age, obese, mother had type 2 diabetes, previous birth of baby over 9 pounds

C. *Pathophysiology of gestational diabetes:* Pancreas is unable to meet demands for increased insulin to compensate for the insulin resistance during the second and third trimesters and maintain normoglycemia.

D. *Identify maternal and fetal/neonatal risks and complications:* See Maternal-fetal risks subsection of Gestational diabetes section. Similar to risks for gestational diabetes except for congenital malformations.

E. *Outline the ongoing assessment:* see Antepartum subsection. Emphasize need for monitoring blood glucose level and urine for ketones, antepartal fetal surveillance, increased frequency of prenatal visits.

F. *State dietary changes:* See Diet subsection. Woman is placed on a standard diabetic diet at 30–35 Kcal/kg for a total 2000 to 2500 Kcal/24 hours.

G. *Implications of GDM:* See Postpartum subsection. Ninety percent of women return to normal glucose levels, but GDM is likely to recur in subsequent pregnancies and there is an increased risk for development of type 2 diabetes later in life. Infant is also more likely to be obese and have DM in the future. Discuss lifestyle changes to lose weight and increase exercise.

5. *Woman with type 2 diabetes unable to take oral hypoglycemic agents:* Inform her that these agents have teratogenic potential; help her to inject her own insulin through teaching, demonstration, practice, and support. See Home Care Box for preparing and injecting insulin.

6. *Pregnant woman with mitral valve stenosis:* See Cardiovascular disorders section.

A. *Need to take heparin instead of coumadin:* See Antepartum subsection.

Explain why an anticoagulant is needed; inform her that coumadin can cross the placenta and harm the fetus, but heparin as a large molecule will not.

B. *Information to ensure safe use of heparin:* routine blood work to check clotting ability; avoid foods high in vitamin K, which inhibits function; discuss alternative sources for folic acid; discuss side effects including unusual bleeding and bruising.

C. *Organic heart disease classification:* symptomatic with increased activity; therapeutic plan. See Antepartum subsection of Plan of care and interventions, focusing on specific measures for Class II; see Teaching Guidelines Box—Pregnant women at risk for cardiac decompensation.

Rest/sleep/activity patterns: Avoid heavy exertion, stop if signs of decompensation occur, get eight to 10 hours of sleep per night with 30 minute naps after meals

Prevention of infection: good hygiene and health habits to maintain resistance, identify early and treat promptly, prophylactic antibiotics

Nutrition: well-balanced diet high in iron and protein, adequate calories, sodium restriction, need for potassium; keep weight gain within limits

Bowel elimination: prevent constipation to avoid valsalva maneuver

D. *Factors increasing stress:* See Assessment and nursing diagnoses subsection of Care management—Cardiovascular disorder section.

Physiologic factors: anemia, infection, edema, constipation

Psychosocial factors: depression, anxiety/fear, financial concerns, anger, impaired social interactions, feelings of inadequacy, cultural expectations, inadequate support system

E/F. *Signs and symptoms of cardiac decompensation:* See Signs of Complications Box—Cardiac Decompensation.

G. 28, 32, hemodynamic changes reach their maximum

H. *Four interventions to prevent cardiac decompensation:* See Teaching Guidelines Box—Pregnant woman at risk for cardiac decompensation.
- Teach about rest, activity limitations, infection prevention, diet to prevent anemia and constipation
- Ensure emotional and psychosocial support from health care provider and support system
- Make referral as needed

I. *Care during labor:* See Intrapartum subsection.
- Comprehensive assessment for decompensation
- Decrease fear and anxiety with one-on-one care and support in a calm atmosphere, keep her informed about what is occurring and how she and her fetus are doing
- Provide pain relief (epidural is recommended); use comfort measures
- Vaginal birth is the best approach from a side-lying position, avoiding Valsalva maneuver, using open glottis pushing with assistance of forceps, oxygen via mask, antibiotic prophylaxis

J. 24, 48: See Nurse alert subsection in Assessment and Nursing Diagnoses section. Problems occur as a result of hemodynamic changes associated with birth of baby and the circulatory and hormonal changes occurring with separation and expulsion of the placenta.

K. *Stress reduction measures during the postpartum period:* See Postpartum subsection. Rest in a side-lying position, assist with ADLs, progressive ambulation, pain relief, measures to prevent infection and constipation, assist with newborn care.

L. *Breastfeeding:* The mother can, but will need extra support due to the increased energy demands associated with breastfeeding.

M. *Discharge planning:* Mobilize support system to help after discharge, make referrals for home care as needed, use time management techniques to plan specific times for activity and rest/sleep, discuss sexuality issues, contraception, and future pregnancies.

7. *Pregnant woman with epilepsy:* See Epilepsy subsection of Neurological disorders section. Inform her that the effects of pregnancy on epilepsy are unpredictable; convulsions may injure her or her fetus and lead to abortion, preterm labor, or separation of the placenta. Medications, which will be given in the lowest therapeutic dose, must be taken to prevent convulsions. Folic acid supplementation is important since anticonvulsants deplete folic acid stores.

8. *Pregnant woman who is HIV positive:* See HIV/AIDS section.
   A. *Care management during each stage of pregnancy:* See Care management subsection.
      Prenatal stage: Assess for drug and alcohol addiction, poor nutrition, concurrent STDs; treat as appropriate; encourage ongoing prenatal care and antepartal testing; support immune system with nutrition, rest, exercise, stress reduction, safer sex; administer AZT, hepatitis B vaccine, PPD test, and prophylactic treatment for pneumocystis; make referrals to drug rehabilitation if appropriate.
      Intrapartum stage: AZT IV to decrease neonatal exposure; keep membranes intact until birth; avoid internal monitoring, use of forceps or vacuum; wipe free of fluids immediately after birth; adhere to infection control and standard precaution guidelines.
      Postpartum stage: Increased risk for infection and hemorrhage; should not breastfeed. Refer for follow-up care.

   B. *Modes of transmission to fetus/newborn:* maternal circulation (prenatal stage), inoculation or ingestion of maternal blood and other body fluids (intrapartum stage), breast milk (postpartum stage)
   C. *Measures to prevent transmission to newborn:* Administer zidovudine (AZT) during pregnancy and labor.

9. *Abuse of drugs and alcohol during pregnancy:* See Substance Abuse section.
   A. *Nurse's approach during first health history interview:* Incorporate questions into overall prenatal history; be matter-of-fact and nonjudgmental; start with questions about over-the-counter drugs, then progress to prescriptions, legal drugs (alcohol), and illegal drugs; screen for STDs; use toxicology screens and questionnaires as appropriate.
   B. *Components and scoring of TACE and TWEAK screening tests:* See Boxes 23-3 and 23-4.
   C. *Factors to consider when planning care and setting outcomes:* See Box 23-5.
      - Consider the characteristics of substance abusers including depression related to negative experiences; abuse may serve as a means of relieving loneliness and emptiness; abusers may have grown up in an environment where abuse is normal and have had little opportunity to learn sober living skills
      - These characteristics can make change and recovery very difficult and interfere with their ability to be caring and nurturing parents; follow-up care is critical
   D. *Nursing measures:*
      - Assist with decreasing then stopping substance abuse; educate about the affects of the substance on the pregnancy and the fetus; be clear and confront if necessary; use the receptivity to change during pregnancy; make referrals for treatment; assess

progress; perform toxicology screens as appropriate

- Recognize that their ability to cope with childbirth may be limited; plan for toxicology screens of the newborn
- Carefully plan for discharge with safety of infant of utmost importance; make arrangements for home visit follow-up, services to help mother to care for baby and continue treatment, and notify child protective services if indicated

Chapter 24: Pregnancy at Risk: Gestational Conditions

Chapter Review Activities

1. *Complete the table related to factors distinguishing hypertensive disorders that occur during pregnancy:* See Table 24-1 and specific subsections for each disorder in the Hypertension in pregnancy section.

2. *Contrast expected physiologic adaptations to pregnancy with those that lead to hypertensive disorders:* See Box 24-2 for a description of normal physiologic adaptations to pregnancy in terms of cardiovascular, hematologic, renal, and endocrine adaptations, and Pathophysiology subsection in Hypertension in pregnancy section for an explanation of ineffective adaptations that lead to hypertensive disorders.

3. *Principles for ensuring accurate blood pressure measurement:* See Protocol Box—Blood Pressure Measurement. Emphasize consistency in position of woman and the arm used, proper size of cuff, and provision of a rest period prior to the measurement.

4. T

5. F

6. T

7. F

8. F

9. F

10. F

11. T

12. T

13. T

14. F

15. F

16. F

17. *Risk factors associated with pregnancy-induced hypertension (PIH):* See Box 24-1 for a list of risk factors including renal and hypertensive disease, family history of PIH, multiple gestation, first pregnancy, maternal age, diabetes, and Rh incompatibility.

18. *Assessment techniques to determine findings associated with PIH:*
    Hyperreflexia and ankle clonus: See Table 24-4, which grades DTR responses, Deep tendon reflexes subsection of Assessment and nursing diagnoses—physical examination section, and Fig. 24-4 *A, B, C* for illustrations regarding performance.
    Proteinuria: See Laboratory Tests subsection of Assessment and nursing diagnoses section.
    Pitting edema: See Physical examination subsection of Assessment and nursing diagnoses section and Fig. 24-3.

19. *Preeclampsia:* effect on fetal well-being
    A. *Describe effect:* See Significance and incidence subsection of Hypertension in pregnancy section. Major effects on

fetus relate to insufficient uteroplacental circulation leading to intrauterine fetal death/perinatal mortality (especially if abruptio placentae occurs), preterm labor and birth, IUGR, acute hypoxia when a convulsion occurs.

B. *Fetal surveillance measures:* See Mild preeclampsia and home care subsection of Plan of care and interventions. Measures can include serial ultrasounds to evaluate fetal growth, NST, BPP, and daily fetal movement counts by the mother.

20. E

21. C

22. B

23. A

24. D

25. *Preeclampsia prevention measures currently being researched:* See Prevention subsection of Plan of care and interventions section for several measures currently being investigated for effectiveness and safety.

26. F

27. F

28. T

29. T

30. T

31. F

32. T

33. T

34. T

35. T

36. F

37. T

38. T

39. spontaneous abortion, incompetent cervix, ectopic pregnancy, hydatidiform mole

40. placenta previa, abruptio placentae, cord insertion and placental variations

41. Abortion, survive outside the uterus, 20, 500 gm, threatened, inevitable, incomplete or complete, missed, septic

42. HCG, gestational sac, ultrasonography

43. internal os, entirely, internal os, incompletely, edge, internal os, lower uterine segment, contract

44. Premature separation of the placenta, detachment, part, all, implantation, couvelaire uterus, clotting defects such as DIC

45. *Disseminated intravascular coagulation (DIC):* See Disseminated intravascular coagulation subsection of Clotting disorders during pregnancy section.
    A. *Predisposing conditions:* abruptio placentae, severe preeclampsia, HELLP syndrome, retained dead fetus syndrome, amniotic fluid embolism, gram negative sepsis
    B. *Pathophysiology of DIC:* pathologic, diffuse clotting that consumes large amounts of clotting factors, leading to widespread external and/or internal bleeding
    C. *Clinical manifestations:* unusual and/or excessive bleeding, abnormal results on clotting studies (Pt, Ptt, platelet count, fibrinogen level, presence of fibrin split products, clot retraction test)
    D. *Nursing care:* careful and thorough assessment, side-lying position, administration of blood/blood products and oxygen, education, emotional support for woman and her family

46. J

47. E

48. H

49. I

50. G

51. A

52. C

53. B

54. D

55. F

56. *Trauma during pregnancy*
    A. *Significance:* See Significance subsection of Trauma during pregnancy section. Statistical data, including incidence, when injuries usually occur, and types of injuries, is fully explained.
    B. *Effects of trauma on pregnancy:* increased incidence of spontaneous abortion, preterm labor and birth, hemorrhage, abruptio placenta, stillbirth, fetal and maternal death
    C. *Effects of trauma on the fetus:* See Etiology subsection. Impact can include death, skull fracture, intracranial hemorrhage.
    D. *Observe for clinical signs of abruptio placenta:* See Etiology subsection. Deformation of the elastic myometrium around the placenta can cause the placenta to separate; signs include uterine tenderness, pain and irritability, contractions, bleeding, leakage of amniotic fluid, change in FHR pattern.

57. resuscitate the woman first, stabilize her condition, fetal, maternal, bleeding, irritability, tenderness, pain, cramps, hypovolemia, FHR, fetal activity, amniotic fluid, fetal cells, primary survey, establish-

ment and maintenance of an airway, ensuring adequate breathing, maintenance of an adequate circulatory volume

58. *Complete TRAUMA table related to priority activity by maternal and fetal team:* See Table 24-1.

59. *Complete table related to infections in terms of treatment measures and nursing considerations:* See Table 24-12.

60. hepatitis A

61. rubella

62. toxoplasmosis

63. cytomegalovirus

64. hepatitis B

65. herpes simplex virus

66. hepatitis C

Critical Thinking Exercises

1. *Woman with mild preeclampsia:* home care
   A. *Signs and symptoms:* See Table 24-2, which differentiates between mild and severe preeclampsia in terms of maternal and fetal effects, and Table 24-3, which lists changes in laboratory values.
   B. *Three priority nursing diagnoses:* See Plan of care—mild preeclampsia home care and Nursing diagnoses subsection. Nursing diagnoses are listed along with several etiological factors including anxiety, ineffective individual/family coping, feelings of powerlessness, altered tissue perfusion, risk for impaired gas exchange, risk for injury to mother or fetus. Altered role performance and altered parenting should also be considered.
   C. *Organization of home care:* See Mild preeclampsia and home care subsections and the Plan of care. Help the couple mobilize their support system,

make referrals to home care if needed, discuss frequency of prenatal visits and antepartal testing.

D. *Teaching regarding assessment of status and signs of worsening condition:* See Table 24-2 and Home Care Box— Assessing and Reporting Signs of Preeclampsia. Discuss signs and put them in writing so couple can refer to them at home; have woman keep a daily diary of her findings, feelings, and concerns; teach family to take a BP, weigh accurately, and whom to call if problems or concerns arise.

E. *Teaching about nutrient and fluid intake:* See Diet subsection and Home Care Box—Nutrition. Emphasize the importance of protein, balance of roughage and fluids, and avoiding foods high in salt and alcohol. Explain rationale for dietary recommendations.

F. *Coping with bedrest:* See Activity restriction subsection, Home Care Box—Coping with Bedrest, and Plan of care. Explain rationale for bedrest/ activity restriction and clarify what this restriction means for her (e.g., how long she can be OOB). Discuss the importance of the side-lying position in bed, relaxation exercises, and diversional activities.

2. *Woman with severe preeclampsia:* hospital care

A. *Signs and symptoms:* Table 24-2 differentiates between mild and severe preeclampsia in terms of maternal and fetal effects; Table 24-3 lists changes in lab values.

B. *Three priority nursing diagnoses:* See Plan of care—severe preeclampsia hospital care and Nursing Diagnoses subsection. Note that altered tissue perfusion, risk for impaired gas exchange, and injury now take on higher priority as the preeclampsia worsens, and her condition in terms of maternal and fetal safety becomes more serious.

C. *Precautionary measures:* See Box 24-3, which lists precautionary measures in terms of the environment, seizures, safety, and emergency medications and equipment.

D. *Administration of magnesium sulfate:* For #1, #2, #3 use Protocol Box—Care of preeclamptic patient receiving magnesium sulfate; for #4 and #5 use Nurse alert in magnesium sulfate subsection of Severe preeclampsia and HELLP syndrome.

(1) *Guidelines:* List guidelines for preparing and administering the medication solution safely; include essential assessment measures that must be completed and documented before and during the infusion.

(2) *Explain expected therapeutic effect:* Discuss what magnesium sulfate is (CNS depressant), why it is given (to prevent convulsions), how it will be given, how she will feel, and what will be done while she is receiving the infusion.

(3) *Maternal-fetal assessments:* VS, FHR pattern, intake and output, urine for protein, DTR and ankle clonus, signs of improvement or worsening condition including signs of an imminent seizure

(4) *Signs of magnesium toxicity:* hyporeflexia, respiratory depression, oliguria, diminished LOC

(5) *Immediate action:* Discontinue the magnesium sulfate infusion, administer calcium gluconate slow IV push over 30 minutes.

E. *Seizure occurs:* See Emergency Box— Eclampsia.

(1) *Nursing measures at onset of convulsions and immediately following:*
- Emphasize importance of maintaining a patent airway, preventing injury, and calling for help
- Document the event and care measures implemented during

and after the seizures observe effects of seizure on maternal-fetal unit

(2) *List problems that can occur:* rupture of membranes, preterm labor and birth, altered LOC, abruptio placentae, fetal distress

F. *Postpartum period recovering from eclampsia:* See Postpartum nursing care of Plan of care and interventions.

- Close and comprehensive assessment with emphasis on signs of hemorrhage (low platelets, DIC, effect of magnesium sulfate), impending seizures, and status of preeclampsia
- Continue hospital precautionary measures
- Continue magnesium sulfate, antihypertensives; pitocin (not methergine or ergotrate, which can increase blood pressure) should be used to contract the uterus
- Provide emotional and psychosocial support for woman and her family; provide time for them to be together and with their baby
- Discuss how her recovery is progressing and the prognosis for the rest of the postpartum period and for future pregnancies

3. *Woman with hyperemesis gravidarum:* See Hyperemesis gravidarum section

A. *Predisposing/etiological factors:* See Etiology subsection, which lists physiologic and psychologic factors including primigravida, maternal age of less than 20 years, obesity, multifetal gestation, hydatidiform mole, ambivalence about pregnancy and parenthood, body change concerns, lifestyle alterations.

B. *Physiologic and psychosocial factors to assess on admission:*

Physiologic: full description of nausea and vomiting, presence of other GI symptoms, relief measures used, weight, vital signs, signs of imbalances, urine check for ketones and specific gravity, CBC, serum electrolytes, liver enzymes, bilirubin levels

Psychosocial: discuss concerns regarding self and pregnancy; assess support system

C. *Two priority nursing diagnoses:* fluid deficit, risk for fetal and maternal injury, anxiety and fear, feelings of powerlessness, ineffective individual and family coping; client's condition will determine the priority, with physiologic diagnoses taking precedence in severe cases

D. *Nursing care measures:* See Hospital care and Home care subsections.

- Discuss measures related to fluid and electrolyte replacement to restore balance; measures to restore ability to retain oral fluids and solids; monitor status to determine readiness for discharge
- Provide psychosocial support for woman and her family referrals to home care, counseling, etc.
- Teach woman about the disorder, how it is treated, its effect on pregnancy and the fetus, and follow-up care

4. *Pregnant woman requiring surgery:* See Surgery during pregnancy section.

A. *Factors complicating diagnosis and treatment:* Enlarged uterus and displaced organs make palpation difficult and change the usual signs and symptoms.

B. *Three common conditions that require surgery:* appendicitis, acute cholecystitis, and gynecologic problems such as ovarian cysts

C. fetus, FHR, uterine contraction, lateral tilt, vena caval compression, fetal, uterine contraction

D. *Discharge planning:* See Home care subsection and Box 24-5. Teach woman and family about what to watch for, care of the incision, activity and rest considerations, and nutrition guidelines for healing.

5. *Woman with ruptured ectopic pregnancy:* See Ectopic pregnancy section.
    A. *Risk factors:* See Incidence and etiology subsection. Include history of STDs, PID, tubal sterilization and surgical reversal of tubal sterilization.
    B. *Assessment findings:* See Signs and symptoms subsection. Findings include missed period, adnexal fullness, tenderness, dull or colicky pain, abnormal bleeding, referred shoulder pain, clinical manifestations of shock.
    C. *Differential diagnosis:* abortion, ruptured corpus luteum cyst, appendicitis, salpingitis, ovarian cyst, torsion of ovary, UTI
    D. Hemorrhage
    E. Methotrexate, destruction/regression
    F. *Two priority nursing diagnoses:* fluid volume deficit, pain, anticipatory grief
    G. *Nursing measures for preoperative and postoperative periods:* See Care management subsection—hospital care. Measures include assessment, general pre- and postoperative measures, fluid replacement, major emphasis on emotional support to facilitate grieving, discussion of impact on future pregnancies, referral for counseling as appropriate, preparation for discharge.

6. *Woman with signs of spontaneous abortion*
    A. *Basis for signs and symptoms:* See Table 24-6; signs and symptoms indicate a threatened abortion.
    B. *Expected care management:* See Table 24-7; includes bedrest, sedation, avoiding stress and orgasm. Follow HCG level with blood testing and ensure integrity of the gestational sac with ultrasound; watch for signs indicative of inevitable abortion.

7. *Woman with signs of spontaneous abortion*
    A. *Basis for signs and symptoms:* See Box 24-4 and Table 24-6. Determine what she means by a lot of bleeding and if she is experiencing any other symptoms related to spontaneous abortion such as cramping.
    B. *Diagnosis of incomplete abortion:* See Table 24-6. Symptoms include heavy, profuse bleeding, severe cramping, passage of tissue, cervical dilatation.
    C. *Nursing diagnosis:* fluid volume deficit related to excessive bleeding secondary to incomplete abortion
    D. *Nursing measures:* See Table 24-7. Measures include prompt termination of pregnancy: assess before and after procedure (D&C), explain the procedure, provide emotional support, and refer for counseling as needed.
    E. *Instructions prior to discharge:* See Home care subsection and Teaching Guidelines Box—Discharge Teaching after Spontaneous Abortion. Advise regarding signs and symptoms of complications such as excessive bleeding and infection, what to expect regarding pain, bleeding, and discharge, measures to prevent complications including hygiene, rest, nutrition.
    F. *Nursing measures for anticipatory grieving:* See Home care subsection and Teaching Guidelines Box—Discharge Teaching after spontaneous abortion. Include time to express feelings, inform her about how she may feel, refer her to support groups/clergy/grief counseling.

8. *Woman with hydatidiform mole (complete):* See Hydatidiform mole section.
    A. *Typical signs and symptoms:* See Signs and symptoms subsection; vaginal bleeding (dark brown or bright red), larger uterus than dates, anemia, excessive nausea and vomiting, abdominal cramps, signs of preeclampsia before 20 weeks gestation.
    B. *Posttreatment instructions:* See Home care subsection; frequent physical and pelvic exams, biweekly measurement of serum HCG until normal for three

weeks, then monthly for six months, then every two months for one year.

C. choriocarcinoma, HCG, uterus

9. *Comparison of a woman with marginal placenta previa to a woman with abruptio placentae, grade II*

A. *Comparison of findings:* Use Placenta previa and Abruptio placentae subsections and Table 24-9 to compare findings for each disorder in terms of amount of bleeding and effects, color of blood, uterine tone, pain and tenderness, and ultrasound findings regarding location of placenta and fetal presentation/position.

B. *Compare management:* Consider home versus hospital care and active versus expectant management for each disorder.

C. *Postpartum considerations:* Potential complications should be the basis for the special postpartum care requirements. Hemorrhage (placentae previa in lower portion of uterus is less able to contract; abruptio placenta has decreased ability to contract because of couvelaire uterus) and infection (lower implantation site, anemia from blood loss) are the major complications related to location of the placenta and the potential for bleeding disorders (abruptio placentae increases risk for DIC); emotional and psychosocial support especially if fetal loss is an outcome

Chapter 25: Labor and Birth at Risk

Chapter Review Activities

1. *Criteria to diagnose abnormal labor patterns:* See Abnormal Labor Patterns section, Table 25-2, and Figures 25-3 and 25-7.

2. *Five factors that cause dystocia:* See Dystocia section. Consider the effect of

- Powers: dysfunctional labor (ineffective uterine contractions or bearing down efforts)
- Passage: altered pelvis
- Passenger: fetal causes related to presentation, position, anomalies, size, number maternal position
- Maternal psychologic responses such as past experiences, preparation, culture, support system
- Maternal position: ability and willingness of the woman to assume a position that facilitates uteroplacental circulation and fetal descent

3. *Comparison of hypertonic and hypotonic uterine dysfunction and inadequate expulsion in terms of causes, effects, patterns of labor, and care management:* See Dysfunctional labor section and Table 25-1.

4. *Postterm pregnancy:* See Postterm pregnancy labor and birth section. *Fill in the Blank:* 42, 294, 10%, inaccurate dating of the pregnancy, irregular ovulatory pattern, estrogen, aging, 37, oligohydramnios, compression

5. *Maternal risks related to postterm pregnancy:* birth of excessively large fetus, dysfunctional labor, lacerations, need to use induction, forceps, vacuum, or cesarean birth, increased anxiety

6. *Fetal/neonatal risks related to postterm pregnancy:* birth trauma and asphyxia from macrosomia, compromising effects of aging placenta, decreased amniotic fluid leading to cord compression

7. *Care management approach related to postterm pregnancy:* assess status of maternal-fetal unit on a regular basis (e.g., daily fetal movement counts, NST, BPP, cervical ripening using Bishop Score); be alert for signs of uteroplacental insufficiency; induction/ripening; support group and continuation of prenatal care; amnioinfusion

8. *Instructions required for woman and family related to postterm pregnancy:* See Home Care Box—Instructions for Self Care—Postterm pregnancy.

9. *Premature rupture of membranes (PROM):* See Premature Rupture of Membranes section. *Fill in the Blank:* amniotic sac, labor, 2%-18%, 24, one week, preterm PROM, prolonged rupture of membranes, unknown, preterm labor, birth, intrauterine infection, compression, prolapse, oligohydramnios, visualization, nitrazine, ferning

10. *Factors associated with PROM:* See Etiologic subsection for several factors including amnionitis, placenta previa, multifetal gestation, malpresentation, polyhydramnios, bacterial reproductive tract infections, maternal smoking

11. *Instructions for home care for a woman with PROM:* See Home Care Box—The Woman with Premature Rupture of Membranes. Emphasize checking for signs and symptoms of infection and labor, daily fetal movement counts, activity restrictions, infection prevention measures including scrupulous genital hygiene, and keeping follow up appointments.

12. F

13. I

14. E

15. D

16. A

17. C

18. G

19. H

20. B

21. *Preterm labor: see Preterm labor section; Fill in the Blanks:* 20th, 37th, demographic, biophysical, behavioral-psychosocial, unknown, 10%, 83%, tocolytic, propranolol (Inderal), calcium gluconate, betamethasone, 34, 24 to 48, side-lying, placental perfusion, cervix

22. *Etiologic factors for each risk category for preterm labor:* See Box 25-1.

23. *Health care and lifestyle measures to prevent onset of preterm labor:* See Plan of care—preterm labor and Protocol Box—Home management of preterm labor. Include assessments required, lifestyle adjustments, and health care measures the woman should be taught to follow. Review instructions verbally and in writing, arrange for contact person the woman can call for concerns between prenatal visits.

24. *Signs of preterm labor:* See Box 25-2 for list of signs in terms of uterine activity, discomfort, and vaginal discharge.

25. *Actions if signs of preterm labor are noted:* Empty bladder, drink three to four glasses of fluid, lie on her side to enhance uteroplacental blood flow to eliminate myometrial hypoxia and decrease uterine activity, continue to count uterine contractions for one hour (if contractions continue at more than four to six per hour she should call her primary health care provider).

26. *Protocol following admission for preterm labor:* bedrest in side-lying position, external monitor, VS, FHR, IV fluids with care, check urine for UTI and toxicology if indicated, sterile speculum examination and test fluid present to determine status of membranes

27. *Maternal-fetal effects of ritodrine:* See Box 25-4 for list of side effects.

28. *Maternal side effects of magnesium sulfate:* Box 25-5 lists side effects for a variety of

body systems; effect on fetus is minimal except indirectly as a result of maternal problems.

29. *Controversy of bedrest:* See Home care subsection of Preterm labor and birth section and Box 25-3. Consider research findings that contrast the adverse effects (maternal physical and psychosocial effects and effects on support system) with proven benefits in improving outcome.

30. *Amniotic fluid embolism (AFE):* See Amniotic fluid embolism section. Amniotic fluid, particles of debris, circulation, pulmonary vessels, respiratory distress, circulatory collapse, 86%, 50%, thick meconium, clogs, DIC, hemorrhage, multiparity, labor, abruptio placentae, oxytocin induction of labor, macrosomia, death, meconium passage

31. *List signs of AFE:* See Emergency Box—Amniotic Fluid Embolism for a list of signs in terms of respiratory distress, circulatory collapse, hemorrhage.

32. *Recommended care management for AFE:* See Emergency Box. Consider interventions

33. *Indications and contraindications for oxytocin induction:* See Oxytocin subsection of Plan of care and interventions—dystocia section.

Crossword puzzle

Across: 1, therapeutic rest; 3, post date; 6, prostaglandins; 9, induction; 11, augmentation; 12, version; 13, failure; 14, breech; 18, magnesium sulfate; 21, arrested; 24, oxytocin; 25, prolapse; 26, protracted; 28, multifetal; 29, hypertonic; 30, prolonged
Down: 1, terbutaline; 2, ritodrine; 3, precipitous; 4, tocolytic; 5, embolism; 7, amniotomy; 8, dysfunctional; 10, cesarean; 12, vacuum assisted; 14, Bishop score; 15, cephalopelvic; 16, hypotonic; 17, propranolol; 19, laminaria; 20, preterm; 22, dystocia; 23, forceps; 27, ripening

Critical Thinking Exercises

1. *Woman with posterior position and difficulty bearing down:* See Dystocia—secondary powers and Table 25-1.
   A. *Identify factors that have a negative effect on bearing down efforts:* amount of analgesia/anesthesia used, exhaustion, maternal position, lack of knowledge about how to bear down, long labor, lack of sleep, inadequate food or fluid intake
   B. *Measures to facilitate bearing down efforts:* Coach her in BDE, help her into an appropriate position (on hands and knees with a posterior position can be very effective), apply counterpressure to her back.
   C. *Recommended positions:* Hands and knees or lateral will facilitate full internal rotation from LOP to OA and prepare head for expulsion.

2. *Emergency cesarean birth:* See Cesarean birth section and Care path.
   A. *Preoperative measures:* Implement typical preoperative care measures as for any major surgery, use a family-centered holistic approach, discuss what will happen, witness an informed consent, assess maternal-fetal unit, insert catheter, start or maintain IV, provide emotional support
   B. *Immediate postoperative assessment measures:* See Immediate postoperative care subsection. Assess for signs of hemorrhage (critical), pain level, respiratory effort, renal function, circulatory status to extremities, emotional status, attachment to newborn.
   C. *Ongoing postoperative care measures:* See Postpartum care subsection, Care path, Home Care Boxes: Pain Relief after Cesarean Birth, Signs of Postpartum Complications after Discharge. Measues include assessment, pain relief, coughing, deep breathing, leg exercises, nutrition (oral and IV). Prepare for discharge, provide emotional

support to deal with disappointment and feelings of failure.

D. *Possibility of vaginal birth after cesarean:* See VBAC subsection. Discuss VBAC and likelihood of its being used since the reason for her primary cesarean may not occur again; discuss possibility of a trial of labor next time and determinations of whether to proceed with vaginal birth.

3. *Fetal position RSA:* See Malpresentation subsection of Dystocia section. RSA indicates a breech presentation; consider that descent may be slower, meconium is often expelled (increasing the danger for aspiration), risk for cord prolapse is increased.

4. *Induction of labor:* See Oxytocin subsection of Plan of care and interventions—dystocia section and Protocol Box—Induction of Labor with Oxytocin.

   A. *Bishop Score—purpose and factors assessed:* See Table 25-3 for factors assessed to determine progress or degree of cervical ripening. Score is used to determine if cervical ripening methods are needed to increase the chances of a successful induction of labor.

   B. *Score of 5 for a nulliparous woman:* Her score should be greater than 9; therefore her cervix will need to be ripened prior to the initiation of the induction.

   C. *Administration of Cervidil:* See Cervical ripening subsection and Home Care Box—Instructions for after Intravaginal Insertion of Prostaglandin Gel for Cervical Ripening.
   - Side effects include vomiting, fever, diarrhea, hyperstimulation with or without fetal distress
   - After administration woman should remain supine with hips elevated for two hours, she may then be allowed to ambulate and be discharged if stable

   - monitor VS, uterine activity, and FHR pattern

   D. *Amniotomy:* See Procedure Box—Assisting with an Amniotomy. Explain what will happen and why, assess before and after procedure, document findings.

   E. *Appropriate "A" or Not Appropriate "NA" actions related to a pitocin induction of labor:*
   (1) A
   (2) A
   (3) A
   (4) NA
   (5) NA
   (6) NA
   (7) A
   (8) NA
   (9) NA
   (10) A
   (11) NA

   F. *Major side effects of pitocin induction:* hyperstimulation, uterine rupture, nonreassuring FHR pattern, water intoxication

   G. *Actions if hyperstimulation occurs:* See Emergency Box—Uterine Hyperstimulation, which lists signs and immediate actions including discontinuing the induction, keeping maintenance IV running, turning on her side, administering oxygen, monitoring responses of maternal fetal unit, and notifying the physician.

5. *Woman experiencing preterm labor discharged to home care:* See Suppression of uterine activity subsection of Preterm labor care management section.

   A. *Instructions for maintaining terbutaline pump:* Discuss use of pump including signs of problems and site care; site change and adjusting settings may be done by woman or by a home care nurse; identify side effects of terbutaline and whom to call if they should appear; teach her how to count her pulse.

B. *Side effects of terbutaline:* See Box 25-4, which lists signs that should be taught to the patient.

C. *Instructions regarding use of the home uterine activity monitor:* See Protocol Box—Home Management of Preterm Labor and Assessment and nursing diagnoses—preterm labor section. Discuss how often to monitor, how to transmit and check results, what to do if contraction patterns indicate resumption of preterm labor.

D. *Coping with bedrest:* See Home Care Boxes—Suggested activities for women on bedrest and Activities for children of women on bedrest. Identify members of her support system and include them in discussions of how bedrest will be managed and how they can help; make referrals to home care agencies if needed.

Chapter 26: Postpartum Complications

Chapter Review Activities

1. Postpartum hemorrhage, Hematocrit, transfusion, uterine atony

2. uterine atony

3. hematoma, perineal, rectal, vagina

4. Inversion of the uterus, hemorrhage, shock, pain, fundal, traction, uterine atony, leiomyoma, placental tissue

5. Subinvolution

6. Shock

7. coagulopathy, idiopathic thrombocytopenic purpura, von Willebrand disease

8. thrombosis, inflammation, obstruction, superficial venous thrombosis, deep venous thrombosis, pulmonary embolism

9. Puerperal infection, fever, two consecutive days, uterus, wounds, breasts, urinary tract, respiratory tract

10. Endometritis, uterine, placental

11. Mastitis, first-time breastfeeding mothers

12. Uterine displacement, posterior displacement

13. uterine prolapse

14. Cystocele

15. Rectocele

16. urinary incontinency, stress incontinence

17. fistula, vesicovaginal fistula, rectovaginal fistula

18. pessary

19. anterior colporrhaphy, posterior colporrhaphy

20. T

21. T

22. F

23. F

24. T

25. F

26. T

27. F

28. F

29. T

30. F

31. F

32. T

33. T

34. F

35. T

36. T

37. T

38. F

39. *List factors increasing risk for specified complications of childbirth:* See Lacerations of the genital tract, Retained placenta, Inversion of the uterus, and Subinvolution of the uterus subsections for full identification of the risk factors for lacerations, hematomas, retained placenta, inversion, and subinvolution of the uterus.

40. *Hemorrhagic shock:* See Emergency Box—Hemorrhagic Shock and Hemorrhagic shock section.

41. *Two-fold focus of medical management for hemorrhagic shock:* Restore circulating blood volume and treat the cause of the hemorrhage.

42. *Four priority nursing interventions for hemorrhagic shock:* See Nursing interventions subsection of Postpartum hemorrhage section; cite interventions related to improving and monitoring tissue perfusion.

43. *Standard of care for hemorrhagic shock:* Provision should be made for the nurse to implement actions independently—policies, procedures, standing orders or protocols and clinical guides should be established by the agency and agreed upon by health care providers; the nurse should never leave the patient alone.

44. *Measures to prevent genital tract infections:* See Home Care Box—Prevention of Genital Tract Infections for a list of measures that should be taught to postpartum women.

45. F

46. T

47. T

48. T

49. F

50. T

51. F

52. *Postpartum depression; Fill in the Blanks:* intense, pervasive sadness, severe, labile mood swings, 10%, 15%, irritability, rejection, jealousy

53. *Predisposing factors for postpartum depression:* See Nurse alert subsection in Assessment and nursing diagnoses—psychologic complications section. Factors include history of mood disorders, meager/absent social support, stressful life events, low self-esteem, poor marital/partner relationship, depressed father, unplanned pregnancy, not breastfeeding, mother or head of household unemployed.

54. *Clinical manifestations for postpartum depression:* See Postpartum depressions without psychotic features section. Manifestations include depressed mood, insomnia/hypersomnia, weight changes, psychomotor retardation or agitation, fatigue, feelings of worthlessness or inappropriate guilt, diminished ability to concentrate, suicidal ideation; at least five of these manifestations must be present every day for a diagnosis to be made. See Box 26-5 for questions to ask to determine if PPD is present and Box 26-6 for a scale to determine the depth of the depression.

55. *Nursing diagnosis: altered parent-infant attachment for postpartum depression:* See Psychiatric hospitalization subsection. Identify measures to reintroduce the mother to her baby, help her meet her baby's needs in a supervised setting, note signs of developing attachment.

56. *Measures to prevent postpartum depression:* See Home Care Box—Activities to Prevent Postpartum Depression for several ideas for interventions and areas for teaching.

57. *Postpartum depression with psychotic features; Fill in the Blanks:* depression, delusions, harming the infant or herself, days, two to three weeks, eight weeks, fatigue, insomnia, restlessness, tearfulness, emotional lability, suspiciousness, confusion, incoherence, irrational statements, obsessive concerns, infant, kill the infant, bipolar disorder, manic, elevated, expansive or irritable

58. *Focuses for care management for a woman with postpartum depression with psychotic features:* See Medical management subsection. Antidepressants and lithium may be given unless the mother is breastfeeding, hospitalization and psychotherapy may be needed, supervised contact with the newborn needs to be arranged.

Critical Thinking Exercises

1. *Postpartum hemorrhage:*
   A. 24 hours, 24 hours, six weeks, uterine atony
   B. *Causative factors:*
      Early postpartum hemorrhage: atony of uterus, prolapse of the uterus into the pelvis
      Late postpartum hemorrhage: subinvolution, unrecognized lacerations of the birth canal, retained placental fragments
   C. *Risk factors for uterine atony:* See Box 26-1. Factors include overstretched uterus related to multiparity, hydramnios, macrosomia or multifetal gestation, traumatic birth, use of magnesium sulfate, rapid or prolonged labor, chorioamnionitis, use of oxytocin for induction or augmentation.
   D. firm massage of the uterine fundus, expression of any clots in the uterus, bladder distension, rapid IV infusion of 20 U of oxytocin, 0.2 mg ergonovine (Ergotrate), methergonovine (Methergine), IM, IV, uterine contractions, prostaglandin$_{F2a}$, IM
   E. *Noninvasive assessments of cardiac output:* See Box 26-2. Include palpate pulses, auscultate heart and lungs, inspect skin, LOC and urinary output, and observe for presence or absence of anxiety, apprehension, restlessness, or disorientation.
   F. *Three nursing diagnoses:* fluid volume deficit, altered tissue perfusion, risk for fluid volume excess, risk for injury, fear/anxiety, risk for altered parent-infant attachment
   G. *List and explain oxytocics used:* See Table 26-1; oxytocin, then Methergine, prostaglandin$_{F2a}$.

2. *Puerperal infection:*
   A. *Predisposing factors:* See Box 26-4. Consider preconception, antepartum, and intrapartum factors.
   B. *Infection prevention measures:* See Home Care Box—Prevention of Genital Tract Infection and Plan of care and interventions subsection of Postpartum infection. Perineal hygiene and measures to maintain high level of wellness are the major focuses.
   C. *Typical signs of endometritis:* See Endometritis subsection. Signs include fever, increased pulse, chills, anorexia, nausea, fatigue and lethargy, pelvic pain, uterine tenderness, foul smelling profuse lochia.

D. *Nursing interventions:* See Plan of care and interventions subsection; assessment, administration of IV antibiotics, supportive care in terms of comfort measures, rest, teaching, provide time for interaction with family and newborn, discharge planning and telephone follow-up.

3. *Mastitis:* See Mastitis subsection of Postpartum infections section.
   A. *Clinical manifestations:* chills, fever, malaise, localized breast tenderness, pain, swelling, redness, axillary adenopathy
   B. *Measures to prevent mastitis:* good breastfeeding teaching and support (especially proper latch on and removal), frequent feedings, avoid missing feedings or abrupt weaning, breast care and early detection and treatment of cracks
   C. *Treatment and teaching measures:* antibiotics, support of breasts, local heat or cold applications, adequate hydration, analgesics, maintain lactation with continued breastfeeding if safe or with breast pumping

4. *Postmenopausal woman with moderate uterine prolapse with cystocele and rectocele:* See Sequelae of childbirth trauma section.
   A. *Clinical manifestations:* See specific subsections.
   B. *Nursing management:* See Plan of care and interventions. Focus on teaching woman about genital hygiene including sitz baths, fluid and dietary measures, how to deal with incontinence of urine and/or stool, and estrogen treatment; be sure that nursing approach used is caring and supportive.
   C. *Safe use of a pessary:* See Fig. 26-11. Emphasize importance of self-care to prevent problems especially related to infection. Instruct woman how to insert and remove pessary to prevent tissue trauma, how to cleanse and store it, use of douching, performance of Kegel exercises.

5. *Woman with postpartum depression:*
   A. *Predisposing factors:* meager social support and stressful life events including recent move to new city, birth, husband busy with new job, bottle-feeding, mother unemployed; mother inexperienced since this is her first baby and she is 35 years of age
   B. *Signs and symptoms:* See PPD without psychotic features subsection.
   C. *Questions to determine depth of postpartum depression:* See Boxes 26-5 and 26-6.
   D. *Measures to help cope with PPD:* See Plan of care and interventions—in home and community subsection. Include husband in discussions and planning, consider relationship with partner and suggest changes and resources they could seek from their church and child-rearing couples in the community; emphasize safety measures for mother and newborn and determine if further care is needed in terms of psychiatric care and psychotropic medications.

Chapter 27: The Newborn at Risk: Problems Related to Gestational Age

Chapter Review Activities

1. preterm/premature

2. term

3. postterm

4. postmature

5. large for gestational age (LGA)

6. appropriate for gestational age (AGA)

7. small for gestational age (SGA)

8. intrauterine growth restriction (IUGR)

9. low birth weight (LBW), less than the expected rate of growth, shortened gestational period, preterm birth, LBW

10. very low birth weight (VLBW)

11. 2500 gm, 37 weeks

12. $\frac{2}{3}$

13. 36 weeks gestation

14. immaturity of organ systems, lack of nutrient reserves

15. *Common causes/risk factors:* Common causes and risk factors for each gestational age problem are identified in the chapter introduction.

16. *Purpose of exogenous surfactant administration:* See Surfactant subsection of Oxygen therapy section. Preterm infant is unable to produce its own surfactant, therefore exogenous surfactant will facilitate alveoli expansion and stability, easing respirations and enhancing gas exchange.

17. *Complete table related to physiologic function and potential problems encountered by the preterm newborn:* Each physiologic function is discussed in its own subsection in the Physiologic assessment section.

18. T

19. T

20. T

21. F

22. F

23. T

24. T

25. F

26. F

27. F

28. T

29. F

30. F

31. T

32. F

33. T

34. *Kangaroo care:* See Kangaroo care subsection in Developmental and emotional care section and Fig. 27-15. Uses skin-to-skin holding to help preterm infants interact with their parents; benefits newborn and parents, increases feelings of being in control, better temperature and oxygen stabilization, fewer episodes of crying, apnea, and periodic breathing, alert and quiet longer, thereby enhancing attachment and development.

35. *Pain in neonates:* See Pain in neonates section.
    A. *Pain assessment in terms of behavioral, physiologic/autonomic, and metabolic responses:* Each type of response is described in separate subsections.
    B. *Pain management strategies:*
       Nonpharmacologic management: swaddling, nonnutritive sucking, distraction
       Pharmacologic management: local and topical anesthesia, opioids, low dose, continuous infusion or intermittent bolus of a narcotic analgesic

36. *RDS:*
   A. pulmonary surfactant, atelectasis, functional residual capacity, ventilation-perfusion, ventilation
   B. tachypnea, grunting, flaring, retractions, cyanosis, breathing, hypercapnia, respiratory, mixed, hypotension, shock, birth, six hours, crackles, poor gas exchange, pallor, accessory muscles, apnea
   C. 72, surfactant
   D. ventilation, oxygenation, exogenous surfactant, neutral thermal

37. C

38. F

39. A

40. D

41. B

42. E

Critical Thinking Exercises

1. *Newborn needing oxygen therapy:* See Oxygen therapy subsection of Plan of care and interventions.
   A. *Criteria to determine need:* increased respiratory effort, respiratory distress with apnea, tachycardia or bradycardia, central cyanosis, PaO_2 less than 60 mm Hg, oxygen saturation less than 92 percent
   B. *Guidelines for safe and effective administration of oxygen:* Observe for signs of complications every one to two hours with pulse oximeter and/or ABGs, controlled oxygen concentration, volume, temperature and humidity, oxygen warm and humidified
   C. *Complete table related to methods:* See specific subsection for each oxygen therapy method.

2. *Weaning process:*
   A. *Signs of readiness:* Signs indicative of respiratory distress are no longer exhibited, ABGs and oxygen saturation are maintained within normal limits, newborn displays adequate respiratory effort without difficulty, good color, improved muscle tone during increased activity.
   B. *Guidelines:* Approach gradually from one method to another with close observation for signs of good or poor tolerance of the change; reassure and keep the parents informed throughout the process of weaning, pointing out signs that their newborn is breathing effectively and is well oxygenated.

3. *Meeting nutritional needs of a preterm infant:* See Nutritional care section and Gavage feeding subsection.
   A. *Documenting assessment findings after each feeding to determine method effectiveness:* Findings include ability to suck and swallow, coordination of each, signs of respiratory distress during the feeding, length of time for the feeding and amount ingested and retained; monitor weight and elimination patterns daily.
   B. 15 percent, two percent, increased stooling or voiding, increased evaporative losses, inadequate volume, incorrect fluid administration, problems with malabsorption
   C. *Procedure to insert gavage tube:* See Procedure Box—Inserting a gavage feeding tube and Fig. 27-7.
   D. *Priority nursing diagnosis:* altered nutrition: less than body requirements related to weak suck associated with premature status
   E. *Principles to follow before, during, and after a gavage feeding:*
      • Measures to prevent aspiration with proper tube insertion, removal, and position check techniques
      • Use breast milk or formula at a rate of 1 ml per hour
      • Cuddle, swaddle infant and involve parents; use nonnutritive sucking

- Assess residual and use residuals as part of the feeding
- Document all findings and specifics of the procedure

F. *Advancing to oral feeding:* Proceed cautiously, checking for gastrointestinal, fluid, and electrolyte signs of tolerance or intolerance for the advancement, decrease gavage feedings as ability to suck is improved.

4. *NICU environment:* See Developmental and emotional care section.

A. *Common stressors:*

Infant stressors: continuous exposure to light and noise; administration of sedatives and pain meds; invasive procedures and medications required for treatment

Family stressors: size and compromised health status of infant, difficult to interact with newborn to make eye-to-eye contact, increased learning needs, concern regarding potential disabilities, fluctuating status of newborn

B. *Cues related to over-stimulation or relaxed state:* See Infant communication subsection.

C. *Measures to provide a balance of stimuli for the newborn:* See Infant stimulation subsection. Measures include water beds, kangaroo care, bundling, coordinated plan of care to provide for period of uninterrupted rest and sleep, pain medications and sedatives as needed; provide diurnal light patterns, decrease noise level, and use stroking, talking, mobiles, decals, music, wind-up toys for stimulation.

D. *Guidelines for positioning:* See Positioning subsection. Consider changing position, preventing aspiration, boundaries, body alignment, sense of security and comfort, teaching parents.

E. *Measures to help family cope with infant's death:* See Anticipatory grief and Loss of infant subsection. Include nursing support during visit to infant, encourage expression of feelings, provide privacy and time to be with the newborn, arrange for memories, facilitate the grieving process, refer to support groups, clergy, and arrange follow-up care.

5. *Parents of a preterm infant:*
   A. (1) B
      (2) C
      (3) A
      (4) B
      (5) A
      (6) C

   B. *Parental tasks:* See Parental adaptation to preterm infant. Tasks include anticipatory grief, accepting failure to give birth to a full-term newborn, resuming process of relating to newborn, learning how their newborn is different, adjusting home environment.

   C. *Nursing measures to facilitate progress through developmental tasks:* See Parental support subsection. Be with parents at first visit, help them to see the infant, explain characteristics, reasons for procedures, encourage expression of feelings, assess their response to the newborn, make referrals to support group and to home care.

6. *Postterm pregnancy:* See Postmature infant section.
   A. *Rationale for increased mortality:* Increased oxygen demands are not met; increased likelihood of impaired gas exchange, leading to hypoxia and passage of meconium into amniotic fluid, which can be aspirated by the newborn into his or her lungs.

   B. *Typical assessment findings:* See Care management subsection for full identification of physical characteristics, including wasted appearance due to loss of subcutaneous fat and muscle mass and peeling skin.

   C. *Two of the most common potential complications:* meconium aspiration syndrome and persistent pulmonary hypertension or persistent fetal circulation; see separate subsection for each complication.

7. *Four major complications in small for gestational age newborn and the rationale for their occurrence:* See separate subsection for each complication in Small for gestational age and intrauterine growth Restriction section; perinatal asphyxia, meconium, hypoglycemia, heat loss.

Chapter 28: The Newborn at Risk: Acquired and Congenital Conditions

Chapter Review Activities

1. T

2. T

3. F

4. F

5. T

6. T

7. F

8. T

9. T

10. F

11. F

12. T

13. F

14. *Physiologic basis for ABO incompatibility:* See ABO subsection of Pathologic jaundice section. Fetal blood type is A, B, or AB and maternal blood type is O; naturally occurring antibodies can cross the placenta, resulting in hemolysis of the fetus/newborn's red blood cells.

15. *Specify events resulting in Rh incompatibility or isoimmunization:* See Rh incompatibility subsection.

16. *Congenital anomalies:* See Congenital anomalies section.
    A. genetic, hereditary, congenital, genetic, environmental, multifactorial, multiple genes, environmental, neural tube defects, congenital heart defects, congenital hip dysplasia, cleft lip, cleft palate, congenital heart defects, neural tube defects, cleft lip, cleft palate, clubfoot, congenital hip dysplasia
    B. *Perinatal diagnosis of congenital anomalies:* See Perinatal diagnosis subsection. Careful observation is essential so immediate care can be provided as appropriate; take note of color, VS including heart and respiratory function, crying, activity level, appearance in terms of structural anomalies such as ears, face, fingers and toes, feet
    C. *Observation of amount of amniotic fluid:* See Perinatal diagnosis subsection. Hydramnios is commonly associated with congenital anomalies; oligohydramnios often indicates renal anomalies.
    D. *Specific types of postnatal tests used for diagnosis of congenital anomalies:* See specific subsections in Postnatal diagnosis section.
    Biochemical tests: PKU, galactosemia, hypothyroidism
    Cytologic studies: chromosomal examination is used to confirm suggestive but not diagnostic clinical appearance
    Dermatoglyphics: study of the pattern of ridges in the skin of the hands and feet (e.g., a simian crease suggestive of Down syndrome)

17. *Congenital heart defects:* See Cardiovascular system anomalies section.
    A. *Maternal factors associated with higher risk:* rubella, alcoholism, diabetes, poor nutrition, age over 40, ingestion of certain medications, use of Accutane
    B. *Four physiologic categories of CHDs and one example of each:*
       • Defects that result in increased pulmonary blood flow
       • Defects that involve decreased pulmonary blood flow and typically result in cyanosis
       • Defects that cause obstruction to blood flow out of the heart
       • Complex cardiac anomalies that involve the flow of mixed saturated and desaturated blood in the heart or great vessels
    C. *Signs that may be exhibited by the newborn at birth indicative of CHD:* weak, muffled or loud and breathless cry, cyanosis unrelieved by oxygen, cyanosis increases when newborn is supine or cries, pallor, mottling on exertion, respiratory signs at rest, activity effects, bradycardia or tachycardia, irregular heart rate, murmurs

18. *Name the congenital disorder:* A, inborn error of metabolism; B, microcephaly; C, hypospadias; epispadias; D, hydrocephalus; E, congenital heart defects; F, talipes equinovarus; G, choanal atresia; H, meningocele; I, omphalocele; J, esophageal atresia; K, anencephaly; L, diaphragmatic hernia; M, myelomeningocele

19. *Birth injuries:* See Birth trauma section.
    A. *Risk factors for trauma:* macrosomia, hydrocephalus, unusual presentations, very long and difficult labor necessitating use of forceps or vacuum
    B. *Signs and treatment of fractured clavical:* See Skeletal injuries subsection.
       Signs: limited use of arm, focal swelling or tenderness, malposition of arm, cries when arm is moved, asymmetric Moro reflex

Treatment: immobilize by fixing arm to body by pinning sleeve of shirt, careful handling when dressing and undressing, supporting bone when carrying and handling, proper alignment

20. T
21. F
22. F
23. T
24. T
25. F
26. T
27. F
28. T
29. F
30. T
31. T
32. T
33. T
34. F
35. F
36. T
37. T
38. F
39. F
40. T
41. F
42. T

43. maternal diabetes, neonatal intensive care, decrease, two to four times higher, blood glucose levels, ketoacidosis, hyperglycemia, glucose, insulin, growth, macrosomia, acidotic, oxygen, carbon dioxide, macrosomia, hypoglycemia, hypocalcemia, hyperbilirubinemia, lung immaturity, glucose

44. *Identifying common cardiac, central nervous system, and musculoskeletal congenital disorders associated with infants of diabetic mothers:* See Congenital anomalies subsection of Neonatal complications section for a full identification of anomalies in each category.

45. *Macrosomic infant with mother who has pregestational diabetes:* See Macrosomia subsection of Neonatal complications section.
    A. *Characteristics:* round face, chubby body, plethoric/flushed complexion, enlarged organs, increased fat (especially around shoulders), placenta and cord are larger
    B. hypoglycemia, hypocalcemia, hyperviscosity, hyperbilirubinemia
    C. *Warning signs of potential complications:* See subsection for each category; birth trauma, asphyxia, RDS, hypoglycemia.
    D. *Infections represented by the acronym TORCH:* See Box 28-1 for infections represented by each letter.

46. *Sepsis:* See Neonatal infections section.
    A. *Complete table related to modes of infection transmission and infection sites:* See Sepsis subsection.
    B. *Risk factors:* See Table 28-3, which lists risk factors according to maternal, intrapartum, and neonatal categories.
    C. *Neonatal signs indicative of sepsis:* See Table 28-4, which lists signs according to body system categories.
    D. *Effective nursing measures for the categories of prevention, cure, and rehabili-*

tation: See appropriate subsection of each of the categories in the Plan of care and interventions section.

Critical Thinking Exercises

1. *Pathologic jaundice:* See Hyperbilirubinemia section.
   A. *Differentiate physiologic from pathologic jaundice in terms of onset, resolution, and bilirubin levels:* See Physiologic and Pathologic subsection.
   B. jaundice, kernicterus
   C. *Explain the underlying physiologic process:* See Hemolytic disorders in the newborn subsection.
   D. *List potential causes for pathologic jaundice:* See Pathologic jaundice subsection.
      Maternal causes: Rh and ABO incompatibility, maternal infections and medical conditions such as diabetes, oxytocin administration, maternal ingestion of certain medications
      Fetal/newborn causes: preterm, LBW, hypothyroidism, polycythemia, intestinal obstruction, cephalhematoma, ecchymosis
   E. *Measures effective in preventing hyperbilirubinemia:* See Plan of care and interventions subsection. Consider the woman whose newborn is at risk and immediately institute appropriate measures such as early feeding, prompt care after birth to decrease stress (i.e., cold stress) and hypoglycemia.
   F. kernicterus, two to six days, hypotonic, lethargic, suck, Moro reflex, high-pitched cry, opisthotonos, spasticity, hyperreflexia, fever, seizures, 24, half

2. *A pregnant woman who is Rh negative:* See Hyperbilirubinemia section.
   A. *Physiologic basis for Rh incompatibility and sensitization:* See Rh incompatibility subsection. If an Rh negative mother's blood comes in contact with the blood of her Rh positive fetus, she will form antibodies against Rh positive

blood which will then be transferred via the placenta to future fetuses. If a fetus is Rh positive, the presence of these antibodies will result in hemolysis of its red blood cells.

B. *Meaning of a positive indirect Coombs' test:* This result indicates that the woman has formed Rh positive antibodies, probably as a result of her spontaneous abortion and not receiving RhoGAM to prevent antibody formation.

C. *Candidate to receive RhoGAM:* Woman is not a candidate because RhoGAM cannot be given once sensitization has occurred.

D. *RhoGAM purpose and use:* Prevents the sensitization; Rh negative mothers who are indirect Coombs negative should receive RhoGAM after an abortion, after specific invasive tests such as amniocentesis and CVS, during the third trimester, and after they give birth to an Rh positive, Coombs negative newborn.

3. *Describe care management of baby born with myelomeningocele:* See Spina bifida subsection of CNS anomalies section. Consider preoperative and postoperative measures, how to position newborn to protect the site, assess neurological function, prevent trauma and infection at the site.

4. *Newborn whose mother is hepatitis B positive:* See Hepatitis B subsection of TORCH Infection section.

A. *Protocol in caring for the newborn:* Hepatitis B immunoglobulin (HBIG) 0.5 ml IM within 12 hours of birth; administer hepatitis B vaccine concurrently at a different site, repeat at one month and six months of age.

B. *Safety of breastfeeding:* It is safe after the infant is cleansed and the vaccine has been administered.

5. *Newborn whose mother had active herpes at the time of birth:* See Herpes simplex virus subsection of TORCH Infections section.

A. *Four modes of transmission:* transplacental, ascending by way of the birth canal, direct contamination during the passage through the birth canal (this is the route for the baby in this situation), and direct transmission to the newborn from infected personnel or family

B. *Clinical signs of active infection in the newborn:* Identify signs suggestive of disseminated infection, encephalitis, and localized infection of skin, eye, or mouth.

C. *Nursing measures for the newborn:* **Care measures for the newborn and parents:** Wear gloves when handling the newborn, inspect for lesions, obtain cultures from mouth, eyes, and lesions as indicated, delay circumcision, discharge with mother if cultures are negative, breastfeeding is allowed if there are no lesions on the breasts, follow-up health care should be arranged. **Vidarabine and Acyclovir therapy:** Use acyclovir at 10mg/kg/day IV every eight hours for at least 14 days to treat infection; use vidarabine ophthalmic ointment for five days to prevent infection.

6. *Newborn whose mother is HIV positive:* See HIV/AIDS subsection of TORCH infections section.

A. *Potential for infant being infected and possible modes of infection:* There is a 20 to 35 percent risk of transmission unless AZT is used. Mode of transmission during pregnancy is transplacental, mode of perinatal transmission is through maternal blood and secretions, and mode of transmission postpartally would be breast milk.

B. positive, three to six months, eight to 15 months

C. *Two opportunistic infections:* lymphoid interstitial pneumonitis, oral candidiasis (thrush) that does not respond to treatment with topical antifungal agents

D. *Average age of onset of opportunistic infection:* three to six months

E. *Care measures for the newborn:* standard precautions to protect infant and health care providers; special care with invasive procedures and care of cord; antimicrobials as indicated for treatment and prevention of infections; counseling, referrals, and follow-up care for testing; immunizations except for oral polio

F. *Safety of breastfeeding:* Since breast milk can contain the virus, the newborn should not be breastfed. Teach the mother how to bottle-feed her baby and demonstrate how she can have close contact with the newborn.

7. *Newborn with thrush:* See Fungal infections section.
   A. *Signs:* white, adherent patches/plaques on mucosa, gums and tongue which bleed when touched
   B. *Modes of transmission:* maternal vaginal infection during birth, person-to-person contact, contaminated hands, bottles, nipples, or other articles
   C. *Management:* infection control measures and good hygiene (including handwashing) to prevent infections; cleanse mouth with sterile water after feeding to wash out residual milk, then instill Nystatin into mouth or swab onto lesions; treat mother's breasts with topical Nystatin.

8. *Newborn with fetal alcohol syndrome (FAS):* See Alcohol subsection for Infants of substance-abusing mothers section.
   A. *Typical characteristics:* See Tables 28-5 and 28-6.
   B. *Long-term effects:* poor attention span, disciplinary problems, learning disabilities, autism, motor, mental and social delays
   C. *Nursing measures:* involve the parents in care of the newborn, encourage attachment, help them create a warm and caring home environment that enhances development, make appropriate referrals to community services

9. *Effect of maternal substance abuse on the newborn:* See Infants of substance-abusing mothers section.
   A. *Signs of withdrawal for heroin and methadone:* See specific subsection for each substance.
   B. *Effects of cocaine exposure:* See Box 28-2 for listing of neonatal effects in terms of physical and behavioral findings.
   C. *Signs of neonatal abstinence syndrome:* Table 28-7 lists signs in terms of GI, CNS, respiratory, vasomotor, and respiratory categories.
   D. *Care management:* Encourage parent participation in care, provide education and social support, maintain nutritional, fluid and electrolyte balance, infection control, respiratory care, swaddling, pharmacologic treatment, referrals, discharge planning.